Challenging the
Road Ahead

by

Dorothy J. Martin

Bloomington, IN  Milton Keynes, UK

authorHOUSE™

First published by AuthorHouse 10/19/2006

ISBN: 1-4208-7460-8 (sc)

Library of Congress Control Number: 2005906791

Printed in the United States of America
Bloomington, Indiana

This book is printed on acid-free paper.

Acknowledgements

I wish there was a way to start and a way to finish acknowledging all those who helped us complete this venture and therefore, helped make this book possible. I don't have room to do that, but there is one God who made each of you and placed each of you in our path, and I thank Him. He is the only one who could foresee Ron and I having the compatibility to even agree to such an undertaking and I thank Him for Ron.

I thank you, Ron, for challenging the arthritis that would not have allowed you to make this trip. I also thank you for being the encourager you have been all of our married lives, during the 1000 mile trek, and while I have been writing this book. Without your patience and support it wouldn't have happened.

Rick and Kathleen, and their family; Brian and Krista and their family; our brothers and sisters, and their families; and our friends, all have helped make this event and this book possible. Even though some of you thought we had gone crazy, you didn't try to discourage us. We thank every one of you for being encouraging or at least neutral. You were never disheartening. I pray that God will bless each of you.

Contents

Introduction

When the idea of walking from Dallas, Texas to Akron, Indiana to celebrate our 50th wedding anniversary was birthed, I had no idea where that trail would lead … our immediate goal was Akron. I still don't know where this trail will take us, but it appears that the journey has just begun. One thing that was accomplished along the roadside was plenty of time to reflect on what my real thoughts about life are.

Then a seed, the germ of an idea, was planted in my mind that I should write a book about our journey … the why and how. As I wrote about our trek through Texas, Oklahoma, Missouri, Illinois, and finally Indiana, many of my personal beliefs surfaced. I share them in hopes that they may encourage you, the reader, to seek your own purpose and joy. I don't expect you to agree with everything I say, but I hope to stimulate and encourage you to think for yourself. Let me share a brief summary here of a couple of my viewpoints:

Our earthly bodies have weight and there is no doubt that they slow us down. Sometimes they hurt beyond endurance; sometimes they refuse to respond to our commands. But my spirit is not entrapped in this body of flesh. As long as my mind is preserved, I refuse to be confined within this armor that I was born into for my earthly travels. I choose to be creative with my mind and I choose to worship my Savior, my God, and find joy in His creation. My prayer is that I can always find a way of being a blessing to others and to Him.

Do not be obsessed with your body and its ailments. Yet maintain your body to the very best of your ability because:

> *What? Know ye not that your body is the temple of the Holy Ghost which is in you, which ye have of God and ye are not your own? For ye are bought with a price; therefore glorify God in your body, and in your spirit, which are God's. (1Cor 6:19, 20)*

Never say, "Why me, Lord?" But let the kid inside you ask the "why" questions often. For instance: "Why do some people call mice, 'rats'?" Is it just because they see them bigger than I do? "Why does a rainbow have streaks of color that goes from side to side rather than up and down?" "And why is it in the shape of an arch?" And if you think you know the answers then ask yourself why you think your answers are true.

You may ask me why I would suggest that you ask "why" questions. My answer is to get you to think outside of yourself and your situations. But why would I find that helpful? I don't know, I'm not really looking for the answers, I just find it fascinating how much I don't know. I am amazed by God and His infinite character reflected in His creation.

My ultimate goal in writing about our adventures of walking through the Midwest is to get you to ask "why" you were created, "what" is your purpose, and "how" are you going to achieve it. And in the end, to seek out the One who has the answers.

Chapter 1
Challenged?

What is a challenge? What are some of the challenges you have faced or are facing? This book is intended to encourage you to become the challenger. The definition of challenge is: a call to engage in a contest or fight. Or another definition is: to call one's bluff. To take it one step forward, let's define bluff. A bluff is a statement or boast designed to mislead or deceive. When we call one's bluff we want them to prove what they are claiming.

I also checked in the Bible for any reference to "challenge." The only instance that I found was in Exodus 22:9. It states:

> *"For all manner of trespass, whether it be for ox, for ass, for sheep, for raiment, or for any manner of lost thing, which another **challengeth** to be his, the cause of both parties shall come before the judges; and whom the judges shall condemn, he shall pay double unto his neighbour."*

In other words, if something has been taken from you and someone states that it is his, you don't need to just fold your arms and concede. Call the bluff!

We hope our story encourages you to challenge the assault on your health and well-being. My husband, Ron, had been diagnosed with disabling arthritis and the dismal prognosis was that he would remain on steroids and arthritis pills for the remainder of his life. The drugs gave him the ability to return to work and maintain a reasonably good quality of life for a person who had just turned sixty-five. But, our concern now was how soon could we anticipate the side effects to kick in and what new challenges would that bring? Ron decided to call the medical bluff.

There is no doubt that the United States has many of the best doctors in the world. However, only a few of them have any education in nutrition. Very little was taught in our medical schools regarding the correlation between diet and disease or the ability of the body to heal itself if given the proper nourishment. It was 1996 before glyconutrient technology was taught in *Harper's Biochemistry* (1996 edition chapter 56) and most of the continuing medical education (CME) hours are provided by pharmaceutical companies. Pharmaceutical companies rarely sell nutritional products or supplements. Nor do they research or teach about them. Your doctor may have received almost no training in this technology.

As you read through this book, you will see that by taking up the challenge, calling the medical bluff, Ron was able to completely eliminate all effects of the arthritis that he had patiently dealt with for nearly 40 years. But not only has he been able to overcome arthritis but both of us reversed symptoms that made us feel our age. We regained our sense of well-being, our ability to dream for the future, and the energy to embark on a 1000 mile hike.

Chapter 2
Texas, Where It All Began

I believe that exercise is important for optimal health but our thousand mile walk was to convince ourselves that the aging process had actually been reversed. Our prayer is that our story will encourage you to take the challenge. I don't suggest that you set a goal to walk one-thousand miles, but a goal to create change by beginning an active role in managing your health, and inserting some adventure in your life.

In October 2003, we were motivated to start a new business that we called Metro Health and Fitness Group. By this time we had not only experienced a new lease on life but had also witnessed others having dramatic improvement in their wellness, once they became active in their quest for renewed health. We were ready for this journey! We had chosen it as a time to raise money for the American Diabetes Association, because our son was diabetic. But our greatest desire was to be an inspiration for others to realize that there can be "life" after a "bad" medical report and to encourage doubters to be bold in attempting what may seem insurmountable. Who knows, you may succeed and if not, try, try again.

In December 2003, our grandson Brant Riner set up a website for us so we could enter a daily diary and pictures of our journey as we went from city to city and town to town. He did a great job and organized places on the site where advertisers could display their businesses, products, and services, to be viewed when anyone entered our site to check our latest news. I thought it was a good idea and Brant, who had finished high school earlier in the year, knew all the ins and outs of creating just what I wanted. Ron and I went to Rochester, Indiana and visited Dr. Laurence Rogers, a former employer of mine. His practice is podiatry and he not only sent us back with bags full of foot care products but heads full of knowledge of what to look for in walking shoes, how to splint a sprained ankle, what to do for athletes foot, fungus, blisters, etc. He was a great encourager. We also talked with Susan and David Haverty, president of *Preview Family Movie and TV Review*, for whom I did bookkeeping. They brainstormed with us about how we could get things done. We were ready to go!

By March 14, we had been interviewed by Sarah Post of the *Dallas Morning News* and had received our business cards. Thorlos® (an athletic sock corporation) had sent us a full supply of running and walking socks, enough for both of us and even more for us to give away on the trip. What a blessing that turned out to be! The only blisters we experienced were when the weather was steamy and my feet got so soaked from perspiration that they actually looked like they had been in the dish water too long. At that point, I had only a very small blister on each little toe. Every day of the trip I was thankful that we maintained good foot health.

On March 15, 2004, Ron and I were in the Target® parking lot at the corner of Coit and Campbell in northern Dallas, Texas. We were joined by my previous employer Elaine Kellam and co-worker Carolyn Roffino, who came out to encourage us on our "lift off." *The Dallas Morning News* photographer was there to get something on film regarding this sixty-six-year-old woman and sixty-seven-year-old man who had challenged themselves to walk 1000 miles to Akron, Indiana, to celebrate their 50th wedding anniversary on July 4, 2004. Our motto and website were the same, www.1000miles100days. com. Could we average ten miles per day through wind, rain, or sultry heat for 100 days? We didn't know, family and friends had serious doubts, and now we had made ourselves vulnerable to the entire Dallas Metroplex (Dallas/Ft. Worth and their surrounding communities).

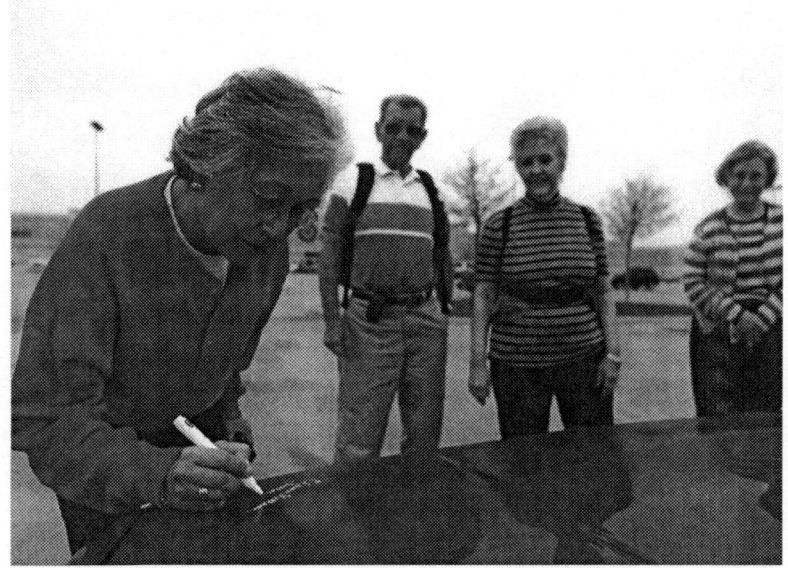

Elaine Kellam and Carolyn Roffino arrived to encourage us as we left from the Target parking lot at Coit and Campbell in Dallas on March 15, 2004. They were first to autograph the hood of Old Red. (Photo by Lawrence Jenkins, compliments of the Dallas Morning News.)

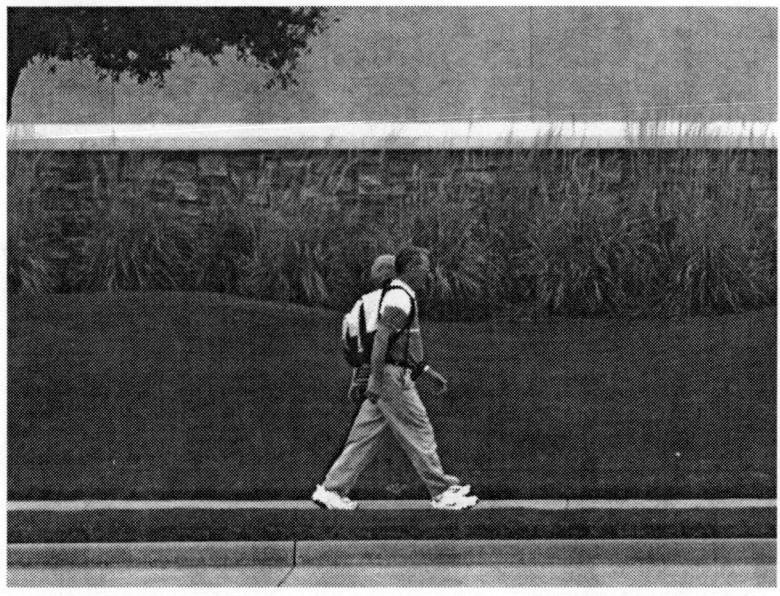

Nearly one mile completed and still walking, stride-for-stride. (Photo by Lawrence Jenkins, compliments of the Dallas Morning News.)

I was exhausted that brisk but sunny morning. Having most recently worked as a bookkeeper, I had resigned from my jobs as of March 1, but I still had to finish my own tax work (since we would be on the road on April 15) and thousands of last minute things before leaving on a four month jaunt. Even through my fatigue, I started this adventure with great joy and lightness of step, excited about this new challenge.

Many have asked us, what would ever possess anyone to undertake such a task. One person even asked me if we were drunk or on something (I think she was teasing). There were many contributing factors: to celebrate the ability to do it after what we thought was going to be a life long struggle with a crippling disease, the adventure, and to raise money for the *American Diabetes Association*. But our overwhelming passion came from the heartache of seeing many people robbed of a decent quality of life long before their productive years should be completed. Our Metro Health and Fitness Group focus is to promote wellness by:

> #1. Peace through faith in Jesus Christ.
> #2. Nutrition and Supplementation.
> #3. Exercise
> #4. Adequate rest.

It has been my nature from early childhood to meet a challenge with a challenge. When I meet individuals who are not finding relief from either spiritual maladies or physical trials, it is my conviction to let them know what has helped me or what I've seen work for others; not that I feel superior, but how can I watch someone hanging by their neck in a rope tied to a tree limb and not even attempt to cut the rope if I think I have a sharp knife in my pocket? It is my opinion that if I say nothing, then I am contributing to their demise.

So, what led us to cook up this trip? It was seeing too many people complacent with where they were, floundering either physically or spiritually, unable or unwilling to commit to change. So, here we were ready to embark on a walk through five states to tell the world that there is hope, don't ever give up!

> *"Hope deferred maketh the heart sick; but when the desire cometh, it is a tree of life." (Proverbs 13:12)*

My hope for this trip nearly faded when we had minimal financial support, in the way of advertising on our website, and had not been able to find anyone to drive our escort vehicle. I was nearly in tears as the last week before our scheduled departure approached. We had secured a loan to meet our expenses, but still no one had come forward to drive for us. I couldn't see any way to walk and drive our support vehicle. But Ron, who is not a visionary but a doer, evaluated the situation and drew up the plan. We would park our car and walk forward two miles, then walk back to the car. We would then drive to our turning point and, if it was in fact two miles, drive forward another two miles. Since we would have walked two miles forward, then two back, we would have walked four miles and we could move the car a total of four miles ahead. Yes, I did get heart sick when I lost hope, thinking we were not going to be able to go forth in this adventure, but when dreams come true at last, life and joy return!

While searching for a driver in local senior centers and churches, I met Jane Steadman who had heard of our need through a church friend. She wasn't offering to drive for us, but she was interested in our trip and had told her Dad about us. Her Dad is Bob Kiser, who has ridden his bicycle from the Pacific Coast to the Atlantic Coast four times. Jane had ridden with him once and the last time he made the trip was in 2003 when he rode with his grandson. At that time, Bob was 79 years old. We felt God was behind this meeting. On the first day of our trip, Bob and his wife Marna were visiting with Jane and he came to meet us as we walked toward Frisco. Jane called on our cell phone to tell us that he was out walking and was hoping to run into us; that we might want to keep a lookout for him. She said that even though he was 79 years old he didn't look like it. It wasn't too long until we saw him. He saw us at about the same time and his long strides toward us gave no inkling of his age. By the time we had walked another seven or eight miles, I was confident that I wanted to know his secrets to youthfulness. His conversation was filled with his love for life and adventure. He gave us a lot of encouragement and a bit of wisdom that stayed with us the full 1,038 miles. He said that for the first few days you will walk on adrenaline. Then as the excitement wears off and you begin to wonder what you committed to, to yourself and to the world, that's when pride won't let you quit, and you'll make it! Bob, Marna, and Jane were our greatest supporters. They had been through the "Are you crazy?" scrutiny and were huge encouragers.

On the second day of our journey, we parked eleven miles ahead of the point where we finished on the first day. Bob and Jane brought us back to our starting point for the day. We backpacked our water and food for the day and any foot supplies that we thought we might need in an emergency.

We were sitting with our feet dangling over an under-the-lane culvert, eating oranges and apples that Bob and Marna delivered to us at about midday, when suddenly I saw headlights about three feet from my back. With the noise of the traffic on the highway, I had not even heard the car pull up. Ron said to me, "Police car." He was sitting next to me and saw it at about the same time that I did. It seems that someone had seen this elderly (I hate to use that word when it refers to me) couple sitting near the road and wondered if there was a problem.

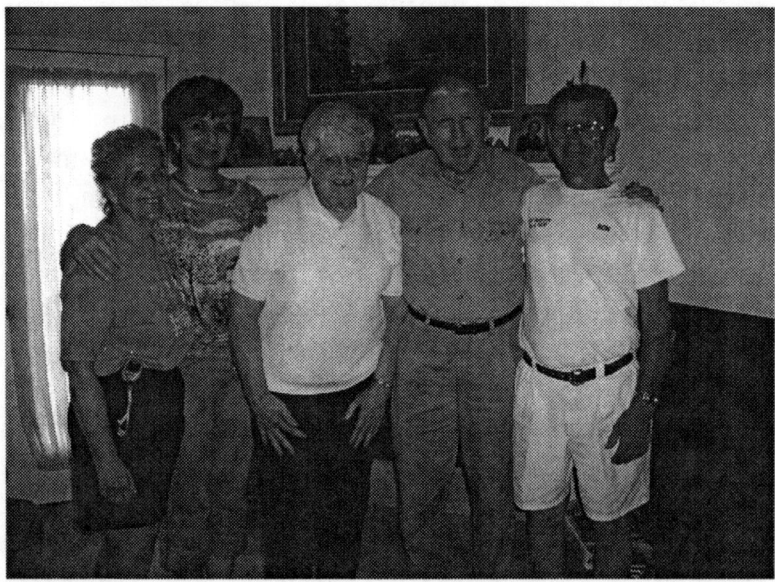

Fun times with Jane Steadman, and her Mom and Dad, Marna and Bob Kiser. (Bob and Jane had ridden bicycles from coast-to-coast. They were our motivators.)

Day three, we were on our own. It didn't take us long to learn that rather than backpacking and walking five to eight miles forward then return for the day, it was much easier to walk two miles forward. Return and move the car four miles, then repeat the procedure. Doing it this way, we did not have to backpack since we were never more than two or three miles from the car.

Our journey through North Texas, via highway 289 which connects North Dallas with Sherman, was a real delight. Being late March, we were ahead of the spring blooming, manicured, roadsides that Texas is noted for. However, everything had the smell of spring; the birds were warbling in anticipation of the coming season of nesting and raising their young. One day, it seemed that a mockingbird followed us most of the morning. I found myself grinning as I pondered if it was really a mockingbird or just a bird, mocking. We had already been mocked by some of our friends and relatives when we announced our plans for the next four months. However, we had one loyal relative who kept up with us and e-mailed us often, our grandson Caleb Riner. I think he thought we were celebrities when he went to *PreviewOnLine* to find the rating of one of the movies he wanted to see and saw our picture and story on the website. (Remember, *Preview* is one of the companies I worked for prior to our journey.) I think Caleb, at the age of thirteen, could still see us as he sees himself. If he wants to do something, he will get it done, one way or another.

It wasn't long until we realized that our religiously followed training of walking through the malls (a great place for winter exercise) had not really given our aging bodies the physical training they needed for the "small" hills and the head winds that we faced on our outdoor hike. However, it gave us a great start and the remainder of the training we needed, we accomplished on the road. As I climbed those hills, I found myself gripping with my toes as I pushed forward. I guess all those barefoot days of my childhood pressed themselves back into my being. Leaning into the turbulent wind, pushing forward with each step, caused my calves to moan, but our spirits were shouting with anticipation of discovery.

On the afternoon of March 19, Ron and I were walking up Texoma (Old Highway 75) in Sherman, Texas. My body was crying for a rest, I think we had walked about nine miles by that time. Ron, however, is like the Energizer Bunny©. Our kids will remember what it was like if you needed a break while traveling. Well, it hadn't changed. Finally, I convinced him that a Chinese restaurant across the street would probably be a good place for a bathroom break, a glass of water, and maybe a couple of egg rolls. As we entered the door, we were met by a gentleman who said that they were closed. Oh, well, Applebee's was next door. My only preference for the Chinese restaurant was because it was closer. The sooner I could get my taxing burden off my feet and onto my shrinking posterior, the more satisfied I was going to be.

Ron showed none of the struggles and fatigue that I felt. I think he had pushed himself through the stiffness and pain of arthritis for so many years that walking ten or fifteen miles through the hills and wind, without pain, for him, was like taking candy from a baby. But let me be the first to tell you, that I would have died before I would have let him complete that walk without me.

We had been in the restaurant a few minutes when a lady came to our table and introduced herself as Dorothy Bishop. She asked if we were the ones she had read about in the Sherman paper, the couple walking to Indiana. We invited her and her husband Bob to join us and spent the next half hour or so visiting over our cool, refreshing drinks and a snack of something that was so unimportant that I don't even remember what it was. This was exactly what we had dreamed our tour would provide, a time to meet new people, to learn about the goodness of the American inhabitants and possibly make new relationships. We were touched by their lives, their thoughtfulness and warm-heartedness, and we hoped that maybe we had inspired them. I returned to the road definitely invigorated!

Before reaching Sherman, we had walked through miles of farm land, areas of little traffic and a view that consisted mostly of flat range land and the curious glances of grazing cattle. After our conversation was exhausted, we had hours for reflection.

Chapter 3
Turning Back the Hands of Time

It was September, 2001, and Ron was suffering accelerated pain from the arthritis that had plagued him for years. In the 1970s he had a calcium deposit removed from his spine. At that time, he lost some strength in his hands, arms, and legs and now it appeared we were headed down the same path again. He was beginning to fall occasionally and his right knee would pop out of socket at any inopportune moment. I wasn't too concerned because with the previous surgery he regained about ninety percent of his original abilities. Since he was turning 65 this month we knew that slowing down was imminent … or was it?

In October, after a complete battery of tests and x-rays, surgery was scheduled. Ron had been "temporarily" placed on steroids and arthritis pills as well as another prescription to protect his stomach from the side effects of the first two. We walked into the hospital to consult with the anesthesiologist regarding preps for the surgery scheduled for the next day. We were met in the hall by Ron's doctor and his anesthesiologist and, as they ushered us into the office, they announced that they had good news and bad news. The good news was that Ron wouldn't be having surgery; the bad news was that they didn't know what was causing the pain and weakness. Their prognosis was he needed to remain on the current prescriptions for the rest of his life. Now, it was my turn to feel weak. I didn't work in a doctor's office for over ten years without learning a few things. Even though the prescriptions gave him the ability to return to work and maintain a somewhat normal life, I had a definite premonition that this was as good as it was going to get ... or was it?

In November, 2001, Ron's follow-up visit had been scheduled. Only one problem, his prescriptions would run out on Wednesday before his appointment the following Monday. I pleaded with the scheduling personnel to reschedule his appointment but was told if he ran into trouble "just bring him to the emergency room." The doctor's office was in the hospital and he refused to renew or extend the prescription until he had an opportunity to meet with Ron. On Friday morning, I called my son-in-law Brian to come and help me get Ron into the car. The evening before, Ron was forced to use both hands to pick up a saltshaker. On this day, once we were able to wrestle him out of bed, he walked in a two-inch, halting shuffle. Brian literally picked him up and put him into the car. After eight hours in the emergency room, armed with a new prescription and an extended appointment date, we were on our way home. Little did we know that this would be our last trip to renew his steroids and arthritis medication.

In August of 2001, before Ron's latest bout started, my brother Dan phoned to tell me about a new science he had heard about called glyconutrients and that there was a food supplement that contained these nutrients. He talked with me about our bodies being able to heal themselves if we supply them with the proper tools, but he said most of us weren't getting some of these "tools" in our modern day diets. He felt it was necessary to add supplements daily.

I had my mother as a guest for four months the previous winter. I agonized with her as she struggled to eat from an over-sized spoon that seemed to be propelled by an earthquake, but actually tossed by the tremors of her Parkinson's disease. It hurt to see her struggle to remember if it was her oldest son who died while she was being held captive by us here in Texas, away from her Indiana home, or if it was her husband's brother. It was her brother-in-law. I was never sure if the confusion was a mental deficiency or caused by the pills she took to relieve the pain of her osteoporosis. Even in my sorrow for her condition, I began to see some of those same traits in myself. I didn't want to go there! Like a drowning person, I desperately grabbed onto the possibility that what Dan told me about glyconutrients was true.

By the time Ron received his diagnosis in September, I was beginning to see a considerable amount of improvement in my own well-being. The involuntary bobbing of my head stopped, "restless leg syndrome" no longer kept me awake at night, and neither did I wake up with leg cramps or inner shaking. I also was able to think more clearly. We decided at that point that it was time for Ron to get serious about a preventative approach, rather than being a complacent "pill-popper." This approach was completely out of character for Ron. He is the original "I can handle it on my own," tough guy. But "his own" wasn't progressing like he wanted; he had gained nearly 20 pounds because of the steroids. In November, 2001, he began taking the glyconutrient supplements religiously and in December, he began slowly decreasing his medications. Before his prescription was completely depleted, he was able to discontinue all prescription drugs. By January of 2002, Ron's knee had completely stopped slipping out of joint. Even though he discontinued his meds in December, 2001, we found that he continued to get stronger and stronger each passing month. Experience made us believers in this nutritional approach to health.

Chapter 4
And God Said:

And God said, "Let there be Ron and Dorothy." And there was Ron and Dorothy. Does that sound egotistical or arrogant? I don't think it is. I believe, as my pastor once said, that God didn't make a child and then decide what His plan was for that child. Instead, He had a mission to complete and made a child to fulfill that task.

Was your life's road paved in gold? Ours was not. Both Ron and I have journeyed down a sometimes dusty, if not dirty path, but God's plan has never changed. Do we know what that plan is? I'm not sure of the details, but today my desire is to encourage you to develop a hope for tomorrow that contains joy and adventure. I believe that when our passion is devoting our lives to helping others, then that passion has come from God.

RON
Even the first day of life was difficult for Ron. He was delivered at home under the attention of the local doctor. It wasn't an easy birth; he was breach (turned sideways in the womb) and by the time he finally made it out into the world, he was beginning to turn blue. Ron was third of eight born to Lewis and Martha Ellen (Sands) Martin ... or was it eleven or twelve?

Ron remembered that he had a sister who was still born and, when his father died at the age of 57, Ron met, for the first time, his half-sister Virginia, born to Lewis and his first wife. Ron's mother gave birth to twin boys when Ron was 14 years old. However, since

Lewis and Martha Ellen were separated at the time of their birth, the twins were placed for adoption. Ron didn't meet them until they were thirty years old. (That's a story for another entire book.) Ron's brothers and sisters include: Ralph, Bob, Charles, Lewis Leroy (Red), and Donald Martin; Virginia Booker, Karen Deeds and Sue Hudkins; plus the twins, Jim and John Fisher.

School was very hard for Ron. Today, I believe he would have been diagnosed with dyslexia, but in those years they knew little about the disorder. He endured the humiliation of not being able to keep up with his class throughout his ten years of school. He eventually quit after his sophomore term when the principal asked him if he was coming back the next school year. When Ron told him, "Yes, I am," the principal responded that he might as well quit, that he was only taking up space, and that this principal would never allow him to graduate. Ron's reply was, "O.K.! I'll quit. But when you leave here, I will come back." However, by the time the principal retired, Ron and I were married and Rick had been born. So Ron was never able to fulfill that promise. Nevertheless, his school experience damaged Ron's self image for life.

DOROTHY

I also came from a big family; born second of eight to Floyd and Jennie (Mills) Koenig. My brother Larry lacked eleven days being one year older than me. The next of the eight was Bonnie, who was nearly five years younger. This meant that, by the time Bonnie was three years old, Larry was nine and I was eight. Since we lived on a farm, the most logical thing to us seemed that if she tried to tag along with us, we promised her we would throw her to the pigs; we didn't have enough time to care for a three-year-old. My brothers and sisters are: Larry, Jack, Dan and Bruce Koenig; and Bonnie Carroll, Carol Koenig, and Kathy Hunt.

Larry was not only my brother but also my best friend. I always laughed, saying that, until I found out that I wasn't a boy, I thought we were brothers. The harsh truth was that I found out way too young that I wasn't a boy. The neighbors of our country home consisted only of boys but, since Larry and I were inseparable, I was always with him and his friends. Before my sixteenth birthday, I had been molested by a teenage neighbor and date raped. When I met Ron, we were both desperately searching for some type of self respect. We reacted much the same way in how we dealt with our self-perceived inferiorities; we both pushed ourselves to excel in life. We set high goals for ourselves, often failing to hit them – which didn't help improve the self-image. Even though we felt like the scum of the earth, we became obsessed with the need to "look" the part of success.

I think Ron was drawn to me because he thought I had what he lacked. I was a top student in school and came from a close knit family. On top of that, I think I might have been considered attractive, even though I felt dirty and ugly. Ron drew me like a magnet. He radiated accepting love … that which I didn't think I deserved to find, and his family always defended each other to the point of arms. Ron loved (and loves) his family. He treated his mother with the greatest respect and helped with the family in any way he could. He displayed what I needed to salve my wounded ego. I felt loved and loved him as much as I knew how, as much as my injured soul would allow.

Did these inferiorities drive us to embark on our journey across the United States to generate news attention? I don't think so. Even though our early-year trials helped mold our characters, I don't think they would have compelled us to exert this type of energy to regain our health. We could not even conceive the thought of such a walk until we regained what was lost, we thought, to aging. I think the early challenges created within us the ability to push beyond the norm, even when others consider us peculiar. But more importantly, I believe they taught us to be compassionate with others who are struggling through their own dilemmas; not only compassion, but a compulsion to want to help them through, to offer hope.

Chapter 5
Oklahoma, The Caring Ones

We crossed the Texas/Oklahoma state line on March 20, 2004. What a day of excitement! With a feeling of accomplishment, we walked up Highway 69 toward Durant, Oklahoma. The next day, as we were moving from our motel in Denison, Texas to one in Durant, I found myself thinking as I was writing in my website diary:

> I have to stop and reflect a bit about the irony of this walk. We are going back to walking the country rather than flying or "flying" the interstates. But the other end of the spectrum puts me in the front seat of my car, typing on my laptop as we drive back to the motel so that all I need to do when I get back (besides packing) is to download my diary update to you. (Just in case you're wondering, I'm not driving, Ron is.)

Oklahoma was a surprise to me in many ways. We had barely gotten into our journey through Oklahoma when a school teacher from Sherman, Texas stopped and introduced himself as Jo Rodgers. He had two bottles of water in hand and told us that the day before, one of his students brought the article about our walk from the newspaper and they had discussed it in class. I don't know what their class discussion was like, but the journal entry I made that day was:

....if I could convey one message it would be, our desire is to attract the attention of as many people as possible ... and especially young people and let you know that it is not about us. We want to inspire you to set some goals, dare to be different! Dare to do what you know will make you feel good about yourself (not to impress others) and I believe that will require you to do something nice for someone else. Go a step beyond the crowd.

We continued up Highway 69 through McAlester and came to the beautiful Lake Eufaula. This lake stretches along the highway for several miles. We walked along its shores for two days. The early morning sun rising to our right, its reflection flashing across the water, and the late afternoon rose, blue, and lavender colors dancing on the gentle waves were breathtaking. In contrast we saw men, women, and children holding their rods and reels, waiting for the big one, as they stood amidst beer bottles, decomposing diapers, soda bottles, bread wrappers, and used tires. We can hope that it was early spring and roadside cleanups had not yet started, but we had to wonder if the fisher folk were part of the cause of this ugly devastation or if they were as dismayed as we were.

We were not far beyond the lake when we met the bravest man in the Midwest. Ron had found another one of his "treasures" that were beginning to fill our trunk. Usually, it would have been a tool or one of those rubber tie downs, but today it was a wicked looking, only slightly rusty, machete - which probably measured about thirty inches long. This was one of those days when the highway was particularly busy, so we were walking single file. When we had to walk single file, I learned to walk in front; otherwise, Ron would stride away, leaving me in his dust. So I will let you visualize this ... I am walking just a couple feet ahead of Ron, who is carrying a thirty-inch machete. If you saw this, what would you be thinking? I'm not sure what my reaction would be, but I'm thinking I would have come nearer to calling the police than stopping to see if help was needed. However, this very nice looking young man, probably in his early twenties, turned his late model vehicle around and stopped near us, as he said, "Just checking to see if you need help."

April 1 was actually a Fools' Day for us. We locked our keys inside the car ... both sets! I'm surprised we had any info about how to call our AARP Road Service. Even though it was our fools' day, it was also our lucky day because Ron had his card in his wallet and a phone in his pocket. We were able to call for assistance. While we were waiting, a couple from Terrell, Texas, stopped to see if we had problems with our car. Once we told them what happened, they stayed and visited for quite a little while as we waited. They also wrote a donation check for the American Diabetes Association. The very next day, guess what tool Ron found along the road! A tool for unlocking locked car doors. Oh well, the day we needed it, it probably would have been locked in the trunk with Ron's other treasures.

One thing that surprised me was in Oklahoma restaurants. In the Dallas area, all restaurants are now smoke-free. However, when we went into the restaurants in Oklahoma, we almost always had to walk through a blue, smoke-filled, room to reach the non-smoking area. Once we got there, it was very likely that we would be the only ones in that section of the restaurant. We heard on the television that the number of smokers, per capita, in the state of Oklahoma was second only to Kentucky. We also heard that Oklahoma had one of the highest obesity rates in the nation. The newscaster's reasoning was that poverty was high in the state. That may also be the reason we found Oklahoma roadways to be the most littered of the states we walked through.

BUT, let me tell you about the people we met in the state. We found Oklahomans were, by far, the quickest to stop and offer to lend a hand. Just seeing our car along the roadway, or us walking somewhere ahead, was enough for many drivers to go to the next crossover, turn around, and come back to see if we needed help. We were often asked if we had car trouble. Every day, we would have as many as ten people stop with offers of aid. Add to that, another three or four police officers pulling along side of us offering assistance or advice. Sometimes we would be advised of areas not to walk through because of crime potential, or highways not to walk on because of restrictions or construction. The news may have reported that the people of Oklahoma were among the most obese in the nation, but we found them to be largest in the area of offering assistance.

Chapter 6
Obesity . . . is it a Cause or a Result of Disease?

I think the answer to this question is like the question, "Which came first, the chicken or the egg?" We know that obesity can cause many diseases like heart problems, diabetes, gout, and many others. However, in my opinion, overeating and obesity may be a disease also, caused by a deficiency. I believe it is very likely that our system lacks the nutrients necessary for maintaining health and vitality. Therefore, it sets up such a ruckus for nutrition that it overrules our reasoning. Like robots, we eat everything set in front of us that can be lifted to our mouths.

Often, the first sign of juvenile diabetes is an uncontrollable craving for sugar. The problem is definitely not eating enough sugar! Sugar is in almost every processed food we buy, especially snacks and soft drinks. The problem is when the body cannot produce insulin or utilize the carbohydrates in sugar for energy, it screams for the carbohydrate deficiency to be met.

With this theory in mind, I advise anyone looking to lose weight to first supplement your diet with necessary nutrients. Many of these needed nutrients are missing in our modern diets. Necessary nutrients may be lacking because of green harvesting, processing and adding preservatives. We have all heard that we need to supplement our meals with vitamins and minerals to "balance" our daily intake. In addition some of the missing nutrients may be the glyconutrients. These are the monosaccharides I mentioned earlier which are necessary for the formation of glycoproteins in the cells. Without these glycoproteins, the cells are unable to communicate properly. Another supplement Ron and I take supplies essential fatty acids. Certain amino acids, found in the proteins we eat, are also needed for good health. I believe you are headed for disappointment if you try to lose weight without making sure that your system is well maintained before, during, and after, your weight loss program.

Would you be willing to lose weight more slowly if you are able to keep it off afterward? If your "diet" is not one that you can live with for the rest of your life, one that provides for a healthy, energetic lifestyle, you are setting yourself up for defeat. Most of us deprive ourselves of necessary nutrition so we can shed pounds quickly. However, if we change our eating habits to maintain what should be our "normal" weight and increase our exercising habits, the extra pounds will eventually come off. Good nutrition for a 125 pound body and increased exercise will not maintain 175 pounds of weight.

Far too many of us want fast results, but when we embark upon a quick weight loss routine by skipping meals and reducing our calorie intake to near nothing, our system goes into "starvation" mode. This means that our body says to itself, "Whoa, we are short of food. Maybe there is a famine." At that point, our metabolism slows down to "save" the stored energy in our fat. In that way the fat can be used more slowly and maintain life longer without food. This is one of the miraculous systems God put into our bodies. The problem (or blessing) is that few of us in the United States have ever experienced a famine. Very few of us need to store extra pounds like we were storing food in the freezer for winter. Most of us have a plentiful supply of food year 'round.

In Dr. Emil Mondoa's book *Sugars that Heal,* he writes:

> *Glyconutrients not only help you lose weight, they help you lose the right kind of weight. In most diets you lose muscle as well as fat, and weight loss is not an accurate indication of fat loss. Your bathroom scale can't tell you if you've lost fat or fat-free mass — fancy words for lean tissue ... Significant lean-tissue loss results in a starvation*

state in which the body actually cannibalizes itself, burning away muscle, heart, liver, and other organs while sparing fat. Anorexia is an extreme example of this phenomenon, which can lead to death.

Exercise is an absolute necessity for both weight loss and good health. You may say that, because of your weight you are unable to exercise. In most cases, that is partially, if not completely, untrue. Anyone beginning a weight loss regimen should consult with their doctor. Do as much exercise as your doctor will permit, or as much as you are physically able (if the doctor will allow you to do more than you are able.) Too often, we think of exercise as some strenuous workout at the gym requiring you to be on your feet. If that kind of exercise is not possible, exercise your arms, do breathing and muscle tightening exercises; consider various forms of resistance training or flexibility stretching exercises. These all help increase your metabolism and your well-being.

Chapter 7
Looking at the Past to Change the Future

In my sixty-five-plus years, I have had the opportunity to see a lot of changes in the United States lifestyle. For the first 55 years of my life, I lived in a farming community in north-central Indiana. I only recall one student, in any of my classes at school, who was overweight and that student had some health issues. I've reflected on my life then in comparison to what I see in today's children.

First, I believe that our food supply was much more wholesome. I don't remember eating anything out of a box, except cereal and crackers. We also ate very little out of a can. The only "canned foods" were in glass jars filled from Daddy's garden. My mother (who we fondly called, Jen) worked hours during the summer, hovering over the pressure cooker, preparing for winter. Our basement shelves were lined with jars of green beans, tomatoes, pickles, peaches, beets, and kraut. The shelves hung over bins filled with potatoes. And we were never without popcorn for our Sunday evening family time, when my mother would continue another chapter or two from one of our favorite novels. We especially liked *Tom Sawyer* or *Old Yeller*. Or we might listen to one of the Sunday night radio stories. Once a month or so, my mother would make chocolate fudge as a treat. Candy or sweet desserts were not common at our house.

Secondly, the fertilizer that was used on our garden was all natural, unlike the chemical fertilizers used today. My father never bought fertilizer. He used what we might call compost. It came straight from the cow barn and horse stalls, was pitched into a pile out side the barn door, and in the spring was spread on the ground. Along with the leftover stubs of plants from the last harvest, the barn manure was tilled into the soil for the next planting. There were no chemicals used for weed control either. Farms were small and what weeds escaped the cultivators were eradicated with the trusty hoe, which also provided a certain amount of exercise.

Farm life had another difference from what we now experience in our urban existence. We never considered starting the day without breakfast. Breakfast often would be served after the cows were milked and the chores finished, at about 7:00 a.m., we never went to school without our morning meal of an egg and toast or cereal. For farmers, the noon meal was normally the largest meal of the day, so we did not go to bed with stuffed stomachs.

Television came into our home during my teen-age years. We had already learned to love being outdoors and wouldn't have found sitting in front of the television all day to be a bit "fun." It would have been more like punishment if we had to stay inside. But most of the early television shows were in the evening and quite often reduced to a "test pattern" after 10 o'clock. What I'm trying to say is that lifestyles have changed and with the changes have come an onslaught of overweight and obese people, along with an outbreak of chronic diseases. Understanding the differences from our past will help us understand what can be done to stem the tide of this epidemic.

I've heard some say that the diseases have been with us all along, but that medical technology had not yet advanced to where they were diagnosed. There is no doubt that the medical advances in this country are beyond my comprehension. However, with all the medical expertise, obesity still rages. Even though science has decreased the number of deaths caused by heart attacks, diabetes and cancer, the number of people contracting these diseases each year continues to rise and obesity can be a contributing factor for all three. Despite the number of diet books in the bookstores and the 24-hour fitness places, I believe the overwhelming presence of obesity is a barometer for the lack of wellness in our country. It appears that eliminating the cause has come in second to suppressing the symptoms.

Dr. Steve Nugent has authored a book titled *How to Survive on a Toxic Planet.* I have heard him say that dietary supplements are no longer a luxury. We are living longer, but, he said, we are also dying longer.

Our medical industry has a great symptom eradication system, but our implementation of a technique for disease prevention stinks. I am thoroughly disgusted with seeing the nauseating ads on TV and on every sports broadcast touting the answer for erectile dysfunction, feminine hygiene, heartburn, athlete's feet or whatever else ails you. Their answer is the newest drug, but if people would check the side effects of their current prescriptions, they may find that a drug is possibly the cause of their problem. I am not suggesting that we discontinue medications without our doctor's advice, but I am suggesting that we ask our doctor about options, a "substitute rather than an additional." Did you know that all drugs have an LD 50 (lethal dosage) rating? Doesn't it make sense that adding another drug with those you already take just increases the potential for further side effects or problems? As you already know, I prefer to substitute nutrition, exercise, rest and relaxation for prescription drugs but, if that doesn't achieve the necessary result, it may be vital to continue your current medicine routine.

There are some that say they do not mind being overweight as medical science has determined. They often comment that being slender is over emphasized and we need to learn to be happy with who we are. While a small percentage may be physically or medically unable to lose weight, far too many use the excuse of positive self-image to avoid changes in their lifestyle. So do we really want to change our standard of living?

Information from the Centers for Disease Control states:

> *During the past 20 years, obesity among adults has risen significantly in the United States. The latest data from the National Center for Health Statistics show that 30 percent of U.S. adults 20 years of age and older – over 60 million people – are obese.*

This increase is not limited to adults. The percentage of young people who are overweight has more than tripled since 1980. Among children and teens aged 6 – 19 years, 16 percent (over 9 million young people) are considered overweight.

These increasing rates raise concern because of their implications for Americans' health. Being overweight or obese increases the risk of many diseases and health conditions, including the following:

- *Hypertension*
- *Dyslipidema (for example, high total cholesterol or high levels of triglycerides)*
- *Type 2 diabetes*
- *Coronary heart disease*
- *Stroke*
- *Gallbladder disease*
- *Osteoarthritis*
- *Sleep apnea and respiratory problems*
- *Some cancers (endometrial, breast, and colon)*

Although one of the national health objectives for the year 2010 is to reduce the prevalence of obesity among adults to less than 15%, current data indicates that the situation is worsening rather than improving.

Now, let me ask you, what could be a reason for you to decide to stay overweight? Are you worth whatever it takes for you to have a happy and healthy life? I don't think that drugs or stomach surgeries are the answers to less disease; maybe a slimmer appearance, but not necessarily a healthier body.

Let me emphasize healthy and happy. I believe it is utterly impossible to be healthy without being happy. Anger, tension, unforgiveness, bitterness and depression all cause oxidative stress. **Oxidative stress causes free radicals, free radicals cause damage to your cells and damaged cells cause disease, premature aging, and many times, obesity.** These are things that you will need to

32

confront, analyze, and find a way to reduce or destroy their power over your mental wellness.

Unforgiveness is spoken about in the Bible with great importance. When Peter asked Jesus how many times he should forgive a brother who sins against him, Jesus replied, *"seventy times seven."* (Matthew 18:21 – 22)   Was this for the benefit of the brother? I don't think so. Mark 11:25 states: *"And when you stand praying, forgive, if you have aught against any...."* What is important about these scriptures is that we do not have the power to ultimately forgive the sin of others and therefore save them from their sin. I believe Jesus did that on the cross. Why we are instructed to forgive them, for what we feel are sins they have committed against us, is for our freedom. Unforgiveness kept inside, in our souls, will destroy us. It will eat at us like a cancer, and the stress of carrying it could eventually trigger a physical cancer or any of a list of diseases.

Here are the steps that will help you take ownership of your weight control program. First, let me remind you that lawyers and the media have blamed the fast food industry for the rise in obesity in our country. I don't believe that. I believe that it is our lack in making quality choices. Here is an example: We have a retirement home in south Texas, so we often go to South Padre Island to spend some time on the beach. When I look at the bathing suits in the shops on the island, I find that about all they sell are thongs. Does that mean that this senior citizen has to buy a thong to wear on the beach? I'll let you decide, but I don't think it is a hard decision.

#1.   Always consult your doctor before beginning any
      weight loss routine.

#2.   Seek to reveal any emotional stress that may cause
      nervous tension and find resolution to those pressures.

#3.   Supplement your diet with nutraceuticals which
      are pharmacy quality nutritional supplements. I
      recommend beginning two to four weeks prior to
      dieting and continuing for a lifetime.

#4. Eat primarily low glycemic foods. There are many good books and websites available that will list these for you. The Glycemic Index lists foods according to how fast they cause the rise of glucose in your blood. The slower the rise of glucose, the less will be stored as fat. Eat sweets in a very limited capacity.

#5. Always eat a light breakfast. It is particularly urgent that you eat only low glycemic foods at this meal. A good rule of thumb is: If you eat fruit, eat if fresh and uncooked. Consume foods that are high in fiber. Stay away from cereals that are sugar coated and avoid adding sugar; a bran cereal sweetened with fresh fruit is a wise choice. Don't use artificial sweeteners or eat fried food. Hash browns are also a poor choice; white potatoes are high glycemic. If you desire toast, choose whole grain bread and use butter sparingly. This meal is very important. Start the day right!

#6. Exercise, exercise, exercise. I know, for most of us, time and energy are important factors in why we don't exercise enough. Remember, if you work in an office, you will need to take a couple of minutes every hour for stretching, tightening and relaxing your muscles, and deep breathing ... yes, that is exercise. Park your car further from the door. Take your children or your dog for a walk when you get home. I like one radio health commentator's advice to "walk the dog even if you don't have a dog." I suggest that everyone wears a pedometer every waking minute. Get one that stores the data for a few days. Each day increase the number of steps from what you walked the previous day.

#7. Laugh a lot!

#8. Get adequate rest. Fatigue has been found to cause cravings for food. Your system is looking for foods that will supply energy. This desire will often show up as a desire for soft drinks or chocolate candy bars which contain both caffeine and sugar. These are definitely not needed when you are trying to lose weight. And, I would say to you, "no diet, caffeine and/or sugar free drinks either." They have absolutely nothing to promote good health!

#9. Drink lots of water to flush toxins that have been stored in your fat cells.

#10. Allow time. Excess weight did not come on overnight and it will not go away overnight, but you may be pleasantly surprised to see it fade away. As you begin nurturing your body, you will gain more energy. As you gain more energy, you will exercise more, and as you exercise more you will, again, gain more energy. As you gain more energy and exercise more, you will lose more fat and acquire more lean muscle.

Reduce your calorie intake to what you will need to maintain your ideal weight; the American Dietetic Association can help you do the math. According to their website www.eatright.org, one pound of body fat equals about 3,500 calories. Reducing your intake by 500 calories for seven days, theoretically, means losing one pound of fat per week. But everyone is different, so weight loss varies. Follow your daily routine of good "balanced" nutrition, exercise and rest. Begin a new lifestyle that will enhance your well-being for the rest of your years.

I have a great concern for those who have reached their goal through nutritional and fitness awareness and implementations. Our medically perceived mindset tends to follow the scenario of a broken arm. After waiting six weeks for the body to heal the break, we take off the cast that was used to assist proper healing. That, of course, is the right thing to do. However, if you have reduced your weight or eliminated disease by a change in lifestyle you will not be able to return to your original patterns and expect to maintain what may have taken you months to achieve. The broken arm was caused by a force, but the obesity or disease was caused by habits, deficiencies, chemical imbalances, environment, or inherent traits. You may find yourself having to begin the process over again. How many of us, myself included, have done that? If you return to previous behaviors, what stops the body from regressing also? Nothing.

Chapter 8
Goodbye, Oklahoma, Already

   While in a motel in McAlester, we met a lady from Minnesota. She was interested in our walk and explained how she motivates herself to ride her stationary bicycle. Of course, she reminded us that the winter in Minnesota is too severe to do much outside walking. Her incentive for her bike ride was to have a map at her side. She would mark where she was starting and where she wanted to go. Then she would ride off the miles. Once she arrived at her destination she would then choose another goal and ride toward it. What a brilliant idea! I may use that to earn a trip to an area I have not yet visited. Once I arrive at the goal on my stationary bike, then I will treat myself with the actual trip. Thanks, Mary, for the inspiration.

   April 4, 2004, was a Sunday and we were in Muskogee, Oklahoma. Ron and I had completed eighty miles of our journey that week, consisting of 189,824 steps along US Highway 69. We looked forward to the Sabbath … the day of rest. We would check the phone book or newspaper for a church in the area where we were staying and attend a worship service on Sunday morning. Even though we didn't walk on that day, we usually did laundry and often used the day to move our possessions to another location up the road.

On this day, we decided to attend a GUTS church. I had heard of this congregation because of the Halloween program they present called "Hell House." Our grandkids have traveled from Texas to Tulsa to attend this production. I've never learned what GUTS stands for, but the name has impressed me to believe that you may need courage to stand for what you believe in ... just what we were feeling. This was a satellite church that met in an old theater in downtown Muskogee, with the service beamed onto the theater screen from the main church in Tulsa.

It was a very friendly, outgoing church with people out helping us park our car and youngsters meeting us before we hardly had the car door open. We were happy to record their enthusiasm and contributions by having them autograph the hood of our car. We started this practice in Dallas. Anyone who contributed to our trip or to the American Diabetes Association was invited to inscribe their autograph with a white paint marker on the bright red hood of our 1996 Ford Crown Victoria. We will remove that hood from the car at some point in time and hang it as a souvenir in our garage or office. It holds a lot of memories.

On Tuesday, April 7, I wrote in our website diary:

Last night we stayed in Pryor. Until this walk I thought that trains were almost a thing of the past but after last night I know that I was wrong. We walked on highway 69 along the train tracks all day yesterday and noticed the number of trains but until our night of rest (or lack of it) we did not realize just how many trains used the tracks across from our room. Since the motel was conveniently located at a crossroad, the long black monster whistled through our room every half hour (Or at least it seemed like it!).We met with a news reporter today and we questioned the number of trains. He told us there was a (electricity) generation plant south of Pryor and the trains carried coal to the plant. During the four hours we walked along the track today we counted five of the noisy beasts and each pulled between 102 to 148 boxcars and most were loaded with coal.

As we were leaving from Dallas we had friends ask if we were going to carry a gun. We didn't think that a gun would be safe in the hands of either of us and we didn't think we would need one. Today was the first day that I remotely wished I had one and that was when a bird on an overhead wire chose to leave his deposit on my arm."

I celebrated my 66th birthday on April 11, 2004, but this year it had special significance over and above the fact that we were in a motel in Vinita, Oklahoma, waiting for the rain to subside so that we could move onward. This day was Easter Sunday. My birthday seemed rather insignificant in comparison to celebrating the resurrection of our Lord Jesus Christ.

We continued on through Vinita, leaving Highway 69 and headed east on Highway 60 and into the country. A little way ahead of us, I saw a field that "contained" a bull and his harem. However, the thing that concerned me was that he was leaning to eat grass along the roadside over a fence that reached only up to his knees. I pointed out to Ron that I thought it might be a good idea to turn around, go back and get the car, and drive past him. Being a country girl in my earlier years, I knew a bull can sometimes get very protective of his "girls." But Ron assured me that it would be O.K. I will admit that Ron was right again, but my vision saw that bull chasing us down the road and I can assure you that Ron can run faster than I … and I thought he would, too.

On the 14th day of April, we came to the Twin Bridges State Park. The countryside was beautiful in northeastern Oklahoma at this time of the year. The roads were lined with flowering dogwood trees and other spring beauty. We had to contemplate how we had lived this long and were still so ignorant of the beauty and assets of our country. An RV park was near the road and bordered the river. We noticed a lot of activity and wanted to stop, but we were somewhat hesitant about taking the time, concerned that we would be late arriving in Akron, Indiana. We had experienced several days during the last couple of weeks when we were not able to average twelve to fourteen miles because of rain.

I quickly recalled some words that I had read earlier that week while lying in a motel room, waiting for the rain to stop. They were written by Peter Jenkins in his book, *A Walk across America,* which recanted his walk in the 1970s. He wrote about mileage craziness. He called it a condition that placed more emphasis on the miles traveled than on the reason for traveling. He warned about being overly concerned with arriving. We stopped.

We watched as boats came to the riverside dock and the passengers displayed their catch. Neither of us had ever seen a spoonbill outside of Sea World. Seeing a fish longer than we were tall, snagged on a hook and line, made us remember the hours we sat on a small lake near our Indiana home to catch a half-dozen six or eight inch bluegills. These anglers said they had only been on the river two or three hours!

We left Oklahoma with many wonderful memories, filled with gratitude for the generosity of the Oklahomans and pictures of the beauty of East Oklahoma burned in our minds.

Chapter 9
The Heartland

On April 15, we entered Missouri at Seneca and by the 20th we were staying in Monett. When the alarm clock clanged about eighteen inches from my tired, snoozing head at six o'clock that morning, I wished I had brought in the sledge hammer Ron had found along the road. First, it was still dark outside. Second, I couldn't reach the light without getting out of bed so I could see how to turn off that siren. Third, my website builder program had crashed the evening before and it was one-thirty in the morning before I finally got everything downloaded and the site information reloaded. But what really irritated me most was the fact that I didn't even set an alarm. We had moved into a new location and I forgot to check the clock!

After silencing the intruder, I went back to sleep and pried my eyes open again about seven-thirty. We wanted to get on the road rather early because the prior evening's forecast called for severe weather starting in the afternoon. I went to the window and peeked out, actually hoping that it was raining so I could crawl back in bed, but the ground was dry. Ron went to the motel office, ate his breakfast and brought a nice red apple and a "small muffin" back for me. I swallowed my fuel, straightened the room a little and picked up a few things to take with us as we plodded on. I was ready to stumble out the door when I heard a rumble ... thunder! I looked out and, you guessed it, it was raining! I could see the water spraying from under the rolling wheels of the semis as they whirred along the highway. I knew now the bed was calling me. I didn't relish having another impromptu shower provided by oily, dirty run-off from the street, splashed by passing cars. It ended up being one-thirty in the afternoon before we got under way for a hike that smelled of spring rains and exposed God's beautiful creation.

While we were in Monett, our glyconutritional food supplements were beginning to run low. We e-mailed an order for enough products to last the remainder of our journey and made arrangements with the motel manager to hold the package for us since we anticipated traveling on to a new location before the shipment arrived. You can imagine our surprise and dismay on April 24 when we arrived to find that the box had been thoroughly destroyed. The packaging looked like it had been run over by a semi or maybe caught in a conveyor belt, and the contents hadn't fared any better. Anyway, our supplies were ruined.

We were so strapped for finances that placing another three hundred fifty dollar order was devastating. But, to keep up our momentum, we felt it was urgent to continue the supplements, especially since we were not getting proper nutrition with our fast food budget. We called our supplier and told them our dilemma. I'm sure they could hear our sigh of relief when they replied, "That's O.K. We will replace your shipment. Where would you like us to mail it?" Whew!

We continued up Highway 60 until we arrived in Springfield, Missouri. From there, we headed north on Highway 65 and by April 27, we arrived at Buffalo, Missouri. This small town, in a rather remote area, turned our technology back a few years. We had neither Internet nor cell phone access … sort of a quiet peacefulness. At the same time, we were concerned that family and friends might become anxious about our lack of communication. From Buffalo, we walked Highway 73 north and turned northeast on Highway 54.

Two days later, April 29, we drove forward in the evening to visit with our grandson, Adam Martin, and his wife, Julie. They were students at the New Tribes Missionary Institute near Camdenton, Missouri, studying to become missionaries in Papua, New Guinea. They originally met in New Guinea during a short term missionary trip. It was good to visit with them and hearing their vision of taking the gospel into distant parts of the world also made us mighty proud. We went back and attended a class on "Church Planting" with them before continuing through the Roach, Missouri area.

At the institute, one of the instructors asked whether we preferred walking uphill or down. By this time, we had encountered some pretty good sized hills. Ron quickly answered, "Up." I was amazed! I couldn't fathom why someone would desire struggling up the rise rather than coasting down it. The instructor said that going up was harder on your endurance, but freewheeling down was much harder on your knees. No wonder my knees were beginning to feel the stress. I had asked Ron a day or two earlier if his knees were feeling any tension and he said, "No." But mine were stiff each morning when I stepped out of bed. I questioned if maybe we would need to discontinue our challenge because it was about promoting health, not destroying it. I also wondered if the distance we had already walked was taking a toll. (By this time we had taken over one million steps.) I was glad to know that the culprit was the downhill slope. The instructor was right, once we got out of the hills, the tightness ended.

Within a couple of days, we arrived at Osage Beach, Missouri and The Lake of the Ozarks. This is another of those beautiful and intriguing places that we were totally in the dark about. I found myself wondering why I had not been more interested in geography; I thought the Ozarks were in Arkansas. I guess we never quit learning!

While in Osage Beach, we attended a church where the gist of the message was, "Working very hard to achieve salvation is similar to being a high jumper. A high jumper in competition, who scarcely nicks the bar and it falls, wins the same prize as the one who doesn't even try." The pastor continued, "The one who works hard to attain salvation has achieved the same reward as the one who doesn't even try. There is only one way to salvation and that is as simple as acknowledging and accepting the ransom and He who paid it on the cross. Works won't do it."

We looked forward each week to attending a different church. Every pastor's message and deliverance was distinctive, however, the warmth or lack of it, radiated throughout the congregation. We witnessed first hand why some churches grow rapidly and why others never grow. Some congregations, we would certainly return to if we moved to the area, others we would not even consider going back a second time.

As we traveled on, we toured the Capital Building in Jefferson City. It contained a museum that visually depicted the colorful history of Missouri. The hand carved lettering over the majestic doorways inside the building was a very inspirational reminder of the principles on which our country was founded. Often something will arouse a song within me and by the end of this day I found myself singing, "I'm proud to be an American, where at least I know I'm free."

Chapter 10
Free Sickness?

If you are not familiar with the term of "free sickness," let me explain what I am referring to. Our American society suggests that everyone should have health and hospital insurance. I am in agreement with that idea. However, here is where the problem lies. We no longer have to be concerned about our health because, if we get sick, we have insurance. It won't cost me anything to get fixed, right? Wrong! If I consider what I hold in my wallet as the only "anything" that it may cost, I could be dead wrong. Yes, it could cost me my life. What has been referred to as "free sickness" is destroying the quality of life for millions of Americans.

There is also the chance that my disease may not be "fixable" with traditional medicine. Perhaps only the symptoms can be managed. Have you noticed how much time a person who has cancer is off work? Or let's think about heart disease, lupus, stroke, multiple sclerosis, fibromyalgia, diabetes, or even "just" the flu or a cold. Does the illness cause you to lose "wallet contents" by purchasing medications and job hours lost? Besides money lost, if I spend the day in bed feeling lousy rather than going to my grandson's football game or band competition, or to my granddaughter's graduation or wedding, then I have lost a part of my life that can never be replaced. Isn't that a significant cost to me?

There are many prescriptions on the market today for the treatment of the diseases that plague our aging population. (As long as we are alive, we are aging.) Many are advertised on the television with the disclaimer, "Ask your doctor if '-----' may be right for you." I am really disturbed by these commercials. In my opinion, they are just a step above advertising cigarettes on a children's program. All medications are hazardous to our health if we do not need them. If your doctor thinks that a certain medicine is the best avenue for your condition, then he/she will prescribe it for you. But, having worked in a doctor's office for several years, I understand that it is almost necessary to give in to the patient's requests, or demands, to avoid lawsuits. I believe pharmaceutical companies are more interested in selling their products than educating physicians about the pros and cons of a drug. Hypochondriac or not, when we see the ads, they may trigger a thought about that symptom and how it would be nice not to have it anymore. But we, who are not trained practitioners, cannot know whether we need the drug badly enough to risk the side effects that may harm our bodies.

I take prescription medicines only when absolutely necessary. Remember, if they are NOT toxic, they are NOT a prescription. Prescription drugs are designed to kill an invading bacteria or virus; or to treat or mask symptoms. And if one drug is toxic by itself, think about taking two or three and in a number of cases even ten or more. If I need a prescription to relieve severe symptoms or make immediate adjustments in my health condition, I will take it. But my goal is to take care of my body by giving it the proper nutrition and exercise in the best way I know how. I discontinue all medications as soon as my doctor will allow.

There is another type of "healthcare" that I have questions about and I hope you will understand my questions. Maybe I just haven't attained the type of faith that some others profess. According to some believers, this healthcare was paid for two thousand years ago on the cross. I believe fully in divine healing and divine health. But I also believe that God provides people (health professionals) to help care for our bodies when they need it. There are many people that teach if we believe in the scriptures, we will live in divine health. We will never need to see a doctor nor be concerned about our health or the well-being of our bodies. They refer to the scripture that states:

Who his own self bare our sins in his own body on the tree;
that we, being dead to sins, should live unto righteousness:
by whose stripes ye were healed. (1Peter 2:24)

This brings questions to my mind. Does that mean we can, "Eat, drink, and be merry?" Does that mean that we do not need to be concerned about nutrition or about supplementing our foods so that our systems have the nutrients needed to heal themselves as God created them? Is it God's responsibility to protect us from the 75,000 new chemicals that we have introduced into our environment since 1930? Are we free from responsibility? If the answer is yes to those questions, then why do we lock our doors when the scripture also states, "*Fear not, for I am with you.*" If God is with me (and I believe He is), why should I have any concern about someone entering my house while I sleep? The scriptures also tell me that if I tithe, my God will *open up the windows of heaven and pour out a blessing* (Malachi 3:10) and in another scripture I am told that "*But my God shall supply all your need according to his riches in glory by Christ Jesus.*" (Philippians 4:19) So why do I go to work?

I believe all these scriptures, but I don't think they free me to abuse the body which God gave me or to live carelessly. After all, scripture also says my body is a temple for the Holy Spirit. I believe that many of our problems in life are due to a lack of accepting responsibility for much of what occurs to us. That brings a story to mind that you may have already heard several times. It goes:

An old man, named Fred, lived in a weather-worn farm house at the bottom of a hill when a heavy rain came down. The water started to rise around his house. A neighbor on the top of the hill saw what was happening and went down with his truck and offered to take the man to his own home until the water subsided. However, Fred replied that he would be O.K. because God would take care of him. So the neighbor drove back up the road to his house on the hill without Fred.

As the water got deeper, Fred climbed his stairs and watched out his upstairs window as the water continued to rise and the rain continued to pour. Now the neighbor on the hill called a rescue group, knowing of the problem Fred was facing. The crew soon arrived in a row boat and asked him to go with them. But Fred was insistent that God would save him. He was not going to go anywhere until God came after him!

The water was now rising much more rapidly so Fred climbed out his window and sat on top of his roof and continued to pray, "Please come and save me." The rescue crew knew that Fred was soon going to be washed away in the torrent so they sent a pilot in a helicopter to get Fred off the roof. But again he refused. As the chopping sound of the helicopter propellers faded away in the distance and the water was now reaching the shingles, Fred, clinging to the chimney on the roof to avoid being swept away by the rain and the wind, yelled out to God, "God! Why are you not answering my prayers? Why have you deserted me? I even witnessed to my neighbor, the men in the boat, and the pilot in the helicopter. I told them I knew you would save me. My faith is strong. I have no doubts. Please, will you save me from this flood, now?"

At that moment there was a flash of lightening, a rumble of thunder, and then a roaring voice from heaven, "Fred, what do you want me to do? I sent a man in a truck, I sent a crew in a rowboat and I sent a pilot in a helicopter. What would you like?"

Author Unknown

God may supply our healing or need through a miracle, a neighbor, a supplement, or a doctor. I believe He will choose the way it will come. In our case, He sent it by way of a food supplement through my brother, Dan.

Are nutritional supplements costly? That depends on what you compare them with. If prevention could save you from losing a limb to diabetes, would you pay whatever it cost? Is there a way to lower the dollar amounts we pay for glyconutrients, vitamins, minerals, EFAs, etc. that we find necessary for maintaining healthy cells? I would encourage you to submit a request to your insurance company for covering nutriceutical wellness products, especially if the company provides a prescription drug addendum. At this time, I don't know of any company that will reimburse subscribers for wellness products. But if we continue to ask, I think the time will come when they will.

Anytime you receive an advertisement for health insurance, I challenge you to write a note on it asking if the company covers wellness supplements. I can assure you that the company wants to insure those who take an active part in maintaining their health. We provide their revenue margin. Insurance is a gamble; we bet on getting sick while the company bets on us staying healthy. If we require less doctor and hospital care, the company gets to keep more of our premium. Why shouldn't they make a provision that covers food supplements, vitamins, minerals, fitness centers, etc. the same as they make a provision for prescription drugs, wheel chairs, crutches, or oxygen equipment? Let's see if we can get it done! Good supplementation isn't cheap as far as money out-of-pocket, but if you consider the alternatives, it doesn't take a rocket scientist to determine a wise choice.

The *Centers for Disease Control* reported that 61% of cancer survivors are age 65 years or older. They estimated that 1 of 6 people over the age of 65 is living with a history of cancer. These statistics highly influence me. They are talking about my age group. But do you know what? Cancer is just one of hundreds of chronic diseases that hinder our elderly from enjoying their later years. Please take heed and enter into a prevention routine NOW.

Chapter 11
The Heart of the Heartland

We trudged northward out of Jefferson City, up Highway 54 through Summit and New Bloomfield. Throughout the lush countryside, I basked in the nature and beauty of God's handiwork. Each step took me deeper into the marvel of God's creative splendor. I don't know why, but road kill surprised me. Some of the distinction of what we saw probably had to do with the time of the year, but there was a definite peculiarity among each state we walked through. In Northern Texas, the primary dead animal we encountered was the foul smelling skunk. Oklahoma's leading flattened species was the armadillo. In Missouri, it was an abundance of turtles. Later, we found Illinois and Indiana to be quite similar with a close race between raccoon and white tailed deer as having been the most misfortunate ones who didn't cross the road safely.

On one day I wrote in my website diary:

Today we saw a small lizard type animal running on the edge of the road. It was very slender and about six inches long. About the last one and one-half inches of its tail was a fluorescent, electric blue and shaded up toward the body into a brilliant purple, then the body was striped lengthwise with what appeared to be brown and tan stripes. I've always been a person who enjoyed touring the pet shops. I'm surprised that if there is an animal with colors this beautiful that it isn't available in the shops. Maybe it is and I just haven't seen it or maybe it has to be in the sunlight to attain those colors, "What is it and why are they not in pet shops?" is my question.

To which my brother Dan replied, "It is probably a Five Lined Skink and the reason that you don't see them in the pet stores is because, if they are caught, their tails usually fall off."

"Yeah, right!" I thought. But a few days ago, our grandson Roc Riner was given a small lizard. It was given to him in a plastic cage. But Roc is not one to be happy just looking at this drab colored animal in a cage. Wouldn't any ten year old want to get a hold of it? (I just happened to be there when this activity took place.) When he put his hand into the cage and started to move it toward this non-descriptive, five-inch long reptile, it began to stomp its small feet. But when Roc was undaunted and closed his hand around the tiny body, about two-inches of tail flew off the main part of that creature and began flipping and gyrating all around the cage while the animal became very still. Well, its God-given defense system certainly worked for him. Roc immediately dropped it in the cage and watched in horror as that tail continued its acrobatic moves for what seemed an eternity … maybe a minute or so, but long enough for the lizard to find cover.

That same day, in the middle of Missouri, I made the following journal entry:

Today seemed to be a day for color. The other dazzling colors I saw had to do with birds, but the problem was that they were all dead along the road. First was the glowing orange and black of the Oriole, the brilliant blue of an Indigo Bunting, the bright blue with a rust/red chest of an Eastern Bluebird, the speckled brown Meadow Lark with the bright yellow breast, and the eye catching red with black mask of the Cardinal. Here is how my mind thinks, "If one of these beauties didn't make it across the highway, what, might I find, in that tall grass, or that woodland over there, or by that stream?"

We were now far enough north of Jefferson City that it was time to look for a new location, so we struck out in search of a motel. As we drove into Fulton, we found all the motels filled because of a work project there. We moved on up the road to Kingdom City and stopped to check for a room. The first one we walked into could not give us a price that would work into our dwindling budget, but they suggested another place. On our way to the offered substitute, we saw a Super 8 Motel and decided to ask there. We enjoyed our stay at one in Neosho, Missouri, so thought we would see what this one could offer us. We were warmly greeted at the front desk by a smiling man with sandy blonde hair, possibly in his 40s, and a blonde-haired lady with a teen-age son. Their names were Keith Johnson, and Cathy and Jeremy Wilkerson. After hearing our story, Keith was able to help us (with agreement from his General Manager, Rhonda Lingenfelter) with a room that was even better than we could have hoped for. Before the evening was over, Keith had arranged a visit from Jamie Lamprecht of KMIZ-TV, ABC channel 17 and Adam Carros of KOMU-TV, NBC channel 8. Both stations were out of Columbia, Missouri. They allowed us to tell our story and promote our fund raising project for the American Diabetes Association on their evening news programs. And, would you believe, Keith also received approval for our entire visit to be complimentary? A free stay was definitely in our budget!

In the heartland of the United States, we found the heart of Missouri. I am very fond of my place of residence in Richardson, Texas. We live in a pleasant neighborhood with good friends and shopping nearby. We are one mile from the area hospital and one mile in the opposite direction from the Senior Center where we go to work out. Richardson is part of the Metropolis of Dallas, so we can attend any of the thousands of things going on there. I anticipate living here for some time. But, if I ever need to move, I hope that maybe Missouri would be the location where I would settle. The hospitality of Calloway County grabbed our affections.

We learned that nearly a month before we arrived in Fulton, Vice President Dick Chaney had been there for a special presentation but, after he left, they decided that maybe he had done too much campaigning on this election year. To even the score, they invited John Kerry. Mr. Kerry had been there just two weeks prior to our visit. I think they were still in the dignitary mode because they rolled out the red carpet for us as well.

Let me tell you about our first day after moving into Kingdom City. Warren Hollrah, a night employee of our Super 8 domicile, met us on our way out and asked us to stop by the Fulton City Hall as we walked through the city. Our hike started just a few miles southwest of Fulton, so we drove back from our motel in Kingdom City to the marker we placed the evening before. Early in our walk, we did a phone interview with Derry Brownfield who is on two hundred and thirty radio stations throughout the Midwest. He had questions like, "If you have to go to the restroom while you are walking, what do you do?" "Look for a tree?" I asked in response. We never revealed the true answer; that would alert passing motorists what to look for.

As we walked into Fulton, we saw the modern architecturally designed building that housed the City Hall. We walked in and told the receptionist that Warren had asked us to stop. She directed us to the office of the City Clerk, Carolyn Laswell. We were surprised to be met by Carolyn and Patrick Bonnot–the assistant to the Director of Administration, Brandi Schubert–a reporter from the Fulton Sun, and the Sun's photographer Alex Hawkey. We were presented with a proclamation which read:

WHEREAS, on July 4, 2004, RON AND DOROTHY
MARTIN, will celebrate their 50th Wedding Anniversary: and

WHEREAS, to celebrate their fifty years together, RON AND DOROTHY MARTIN have decided to walk from their home in Richardson, Texas to Akron, Indiana to benefit the American Diabetes Association: and

WHEREAS, their life together has been one of service to their family and community, we are pleased to join in extending our best wishes to the Martin's as they visit the Kingdom of Callaway and the City of Fulton, Missouri.

IN WITNESS WHEREOF, I do hereby cause the Seal of the City of Fulton to be affixed on this 10th day of May, 2004.

Robert W Craghead
Mayor

ATTEST:

Carolyn L. Laswell, CMC
City Clerk

Not only did they extend their best wishes but also their hospitality! We received souvenirs; sun catchers of the historical City Hall of Fulton, key chains noting the establishment of Callaway County in 1820, and commemorative coins of the Winston Churchill Memorial. Then we were guests of our night clerk Warren for soup, sandwich, and salad at the Court Street Coffee and met him later at the Auto World Car Museum where he works days. This museum displayed the personal collection of William E. Backer. Hundreds of vintage vehicles and antiquated memorabilia filled the area and brought back nostalgic memories.

After finishing twelve and one-half miles on the streets in and near Fulton, we were met by Warren who then took us to meet Coach and Olympic Medalist, Richard Ault and his wife Barbara. Dick was a medalist in the 1948 Olympics in the 400 meter hurdles and went on to set the world record in 1949. (We hope to go back to visit with this couple again.) After visiting with Dick and Barbara, we toured some of the local historical sites, including the Churchill Memorial, and a portion of the Berlin Wall. While Warren was showing us around Fulton, Keith was back at the motel raising money for the American Diabetes Association. He also arranged for our complimentary dinner at the Iron Skillet. By the time we showered, updated our website diary, and crashed into bed, this aged couple collapsed, exhausted and enamored by the Show Me State and its citizens.

Before we left Kingdom City, Warren took us to radio station KFAL where we were talk show guests of Jeremy Washington. Let me tell you something about Ron. Ron is, more often than not, quiet in crowds; even in groups of only three or four people. Occasionally, however, there is someone who can draw Ron out of his shell. Jeremy was one of those persons. However, when that happens, no one knows what will come out of Ron's mouth. He had Jeremy and Warren rolling with laughter, but I was cringing, wondering what Ron was going to tell next. He even told secrets we didn't have … in other words, when he's entertaining, Ron doesn't always stick real close to the truth. For anyone who might have heard the interview, he really didn't have to tie a rope to me to keep me from walking too slow. Nor did he have to tell the whole listening populace that we got married on the 4th of July because of possible fireworks; my Dad's shotgun. The good thing is that he tells such wild stories, no one knows if any of it's true. It was a fun time.

Warren also introduced us to Todd Winterbower, Executive Director of the Heart of Missouri Tourism Center & Fire Fighters Memorial of Missouri in Kingdom City. Todd gifted both of us with a T-shirt and informative brochures about the Center and the area; we then attended a campaign speech by Matt Blunt, Secretary of State of Missouri at that time. Blunt has since been elected governor. He autographed a book given us by Warren and had his picture taken with Ron. We were guests of Keith and Cathy for dinner at the El Vaquero Mexican Restaurant in Mexico, Missouri; Brian Corcoran of KWWR radio station in Mexico interviewed us; Ryan Smith of The Mexico Ledger published a nice article about our trip with a photograph by Brenda Fike; John Sullivan, reporter with the Columbia News, and its photographer, Ed Pfueller, walked with us a couple of miles one day while getting data for their report. Our original greeter, Keith, raised $218.50 for our American Diabetes Association campaign and Rhonda arranged with manager Spike Ehrhardt for our visit to the Super 8 Motel in Bowling Green, Missouri to be free as well. What a whirlwind!

We were immensely impressed with the connectivity among the people in Callaway County and the surrounding area. They seemed to have a close network of contacts and each portrayed a genuine concern for these visitors from Texas. We will never forget the heart of Missouri.

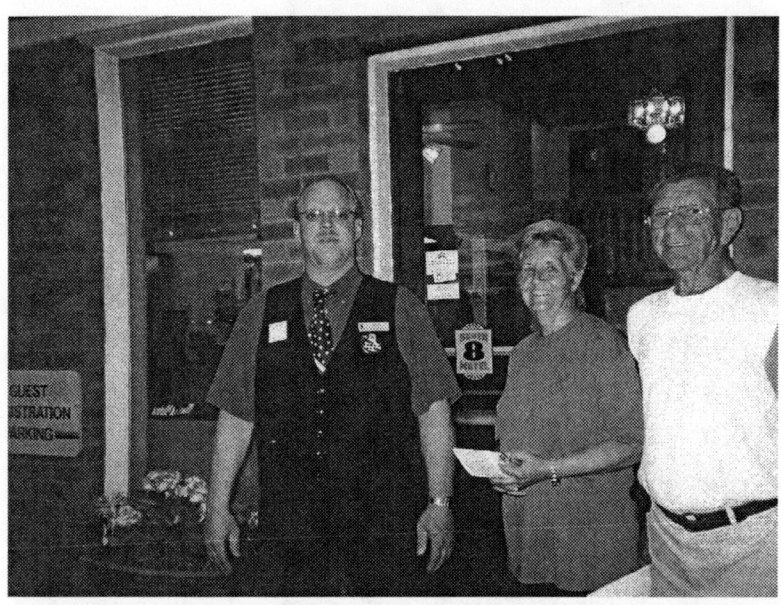

Keith Johnson was our one-man promoter and, without him, this adventure would not have been the same. We consider him one of the angels we met along the way.

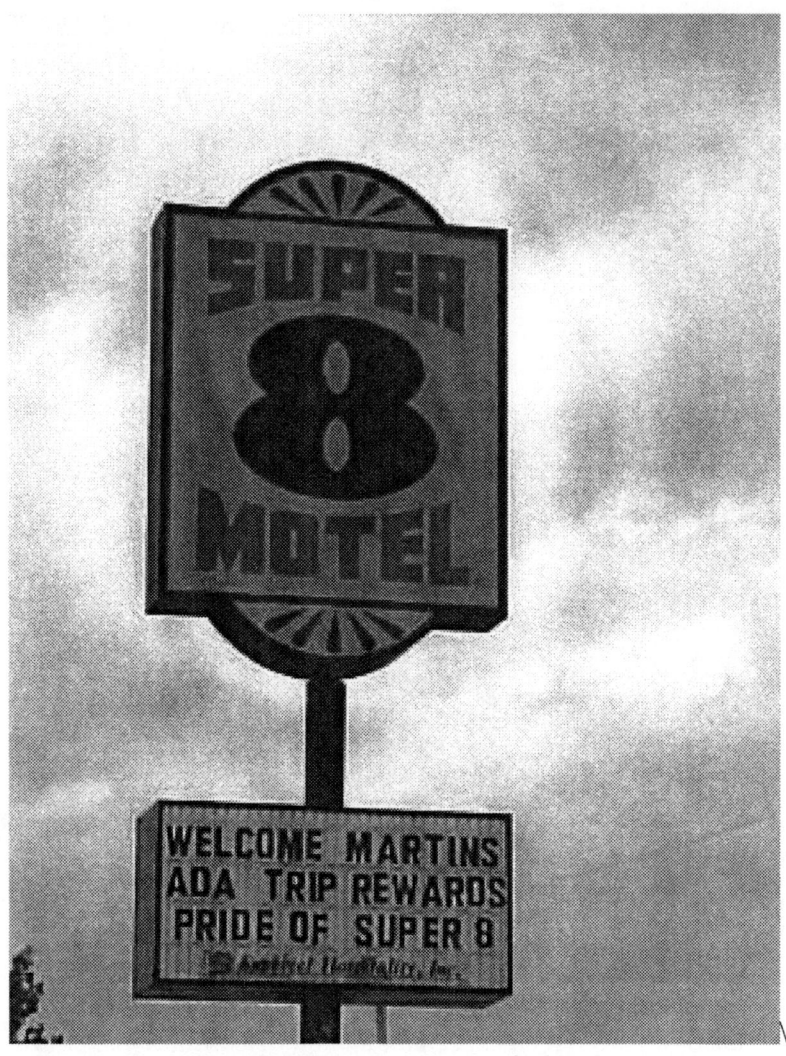

We weren't expecting to see our name in lights, but it was nice.

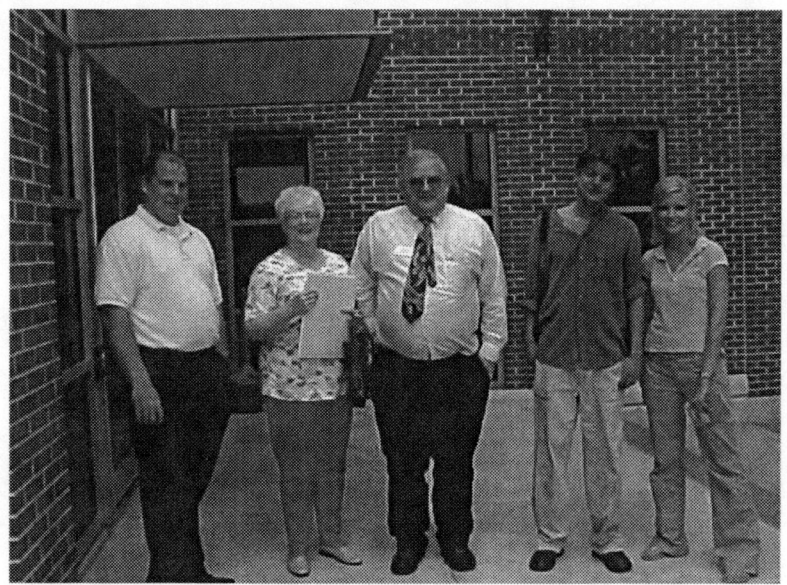

Patrick Bonnot and Carolyn Laswell from the Fulton City Hall; Warren Hollrah, our new friend and tour guide; photographer Alex Hawkey, and reporter Brandi Schubert of the Fulton (MO) Sun.

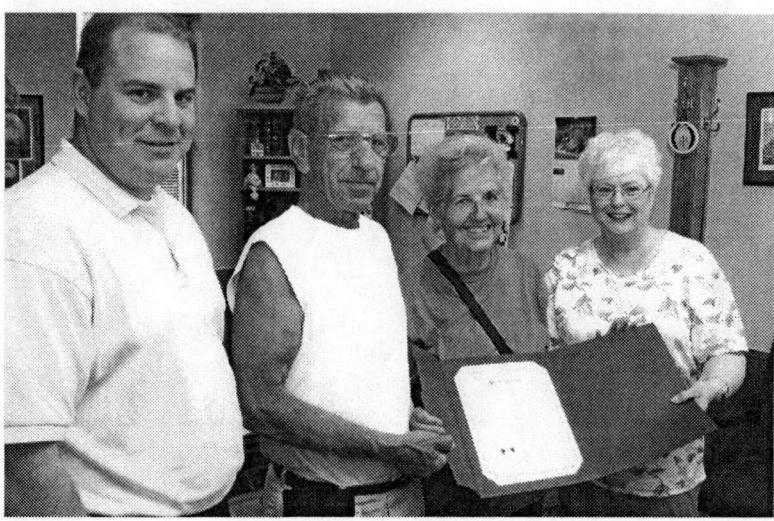

Patrick Bonnot and Carolyn Laswell presenting Ron and I with a proclamation from the City of Fulton during our visit at City Hall. (Photo by Alex Hawkey and compliments of the Fulton [MO] Sun)

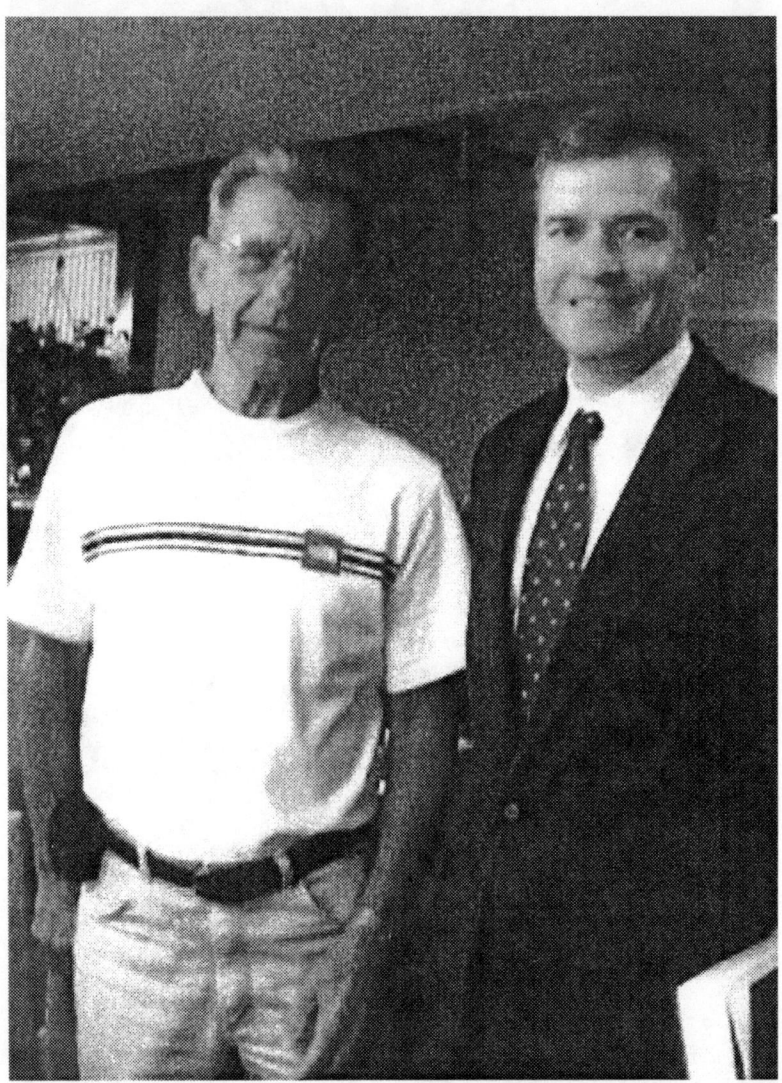

While attending the campaign speech, Ron posed with Matt Blunt, the Missouri Secretary of State and Governor hopeful. (Mr. Blunt has since been elected Governor of the state of Missouri.)

Chapter 12
The Face of People

By May 15, two months after leaving Dallas, we were leaving Calloway County, Missouri, and heading northeast on Highway 54 toward Bowling Green. There, we would turn north on Highway 81 and head toward Hannibal and cross the Mississippi River into Illinois. It was Saturday and morning found us in the small town of Vandalia. As we walked down the tree-lined street in the warm, quiet surroundings, we were met by two boys on bicycles. The boys may have been about junior high age and one of them acted as the spokesperson. He almost seemed like one of the reporters we had met along the way. Later we learned that his name was Jay, actually his name was a longer version of Jay but since I was badly mangling the spelling and pronunciation, he told us that his friends just call him Jay. Jay began to interrogate us: "Are you walking for Diabetes?" "Yes." "Do you have diabetes?" "No, but our son does." "Can people give money to you for diabetes?" "Yes." "Can I give you money?" My first instinct was to answer no because of his age. But then I quickly considered his caring and giving character and replied, "Yes." He reached into his pocket and pulled out $1.75 and offered it as his contribution.

I was touched, almost to the point of tears, but also perplexed. How did this young man know all this? I looked at him, a little bewildered, and as I stared, I had a flashback of an older pick-up truck that had stopped the evening before to see if we needed help. It was traveling in the same direction we were, so it came to a halt across the road from us. Ron walked across the street to talk with them and thank them for their offer of assistance. I watched from the far side of the road. What I saw in the truck was a man driving with two or three children with him. I saw the round face of one of the boys as he watched Ron intently and seemed to hang on every word he was saying. "Jay, were you in that pick-up truck that stopped last evening to see if we needed help?" His reply was yes. What a testimony for my belief that children learn what they see. This young man had witnessed a father, or maybe a relative, who took his time to stop and offer assistance to a couple of strangers. The very next day, Jay presented what he could to the same couple of strangers.

After leaving Bowling Green, we went to Hannibal in search of a motel for our headquarters during our next three or four days of walking. As I mentioned before, we usually inquired at independent lodging locations because of our need to minimize expenses. In Hannibal, we stopped at a small motel that looked somewhat questionable. When we entered the office, we found it empty. We tapped the bell and within a short time were met by a somewhat overweight, young lady, maybe in her late twenties.

She appeared to be groggy but, when we asked the price of the room, she quoted a fee that was within our range. We asked if we could see the room. We told her we were walking for the American Diabetes Association, at which she responded that she was bi-polar. As she walked around the desk, I was astounded! She was bare-foot and had what appeared to be dried blood on her hands. It also seemed to be on the back of her legs and had dripped down and dried on her heels. I was still trying to process this in my mind when we arrived at the room. It was about five-thirty in the afternoon. We walked into a dimly lit "suite" where we apparently disturbed a burly looking man who was cleaning. He proceeded to put a "fresh" sheet on the bed, but his wide, glaring eyes never left us. Before making a decision about a place to stay, we always checked the bathroom for mildew and cleanliness. I don't know if I even looked. I knew I could not leave that place quick enough. Even to this day, I cannot think of any logical reason for what we saw, but neither did we report it to the police. I still wonder if we should have.

Hannibal is a beautiful tourist location which displays many attractions and exhibits about Mark Twain. Samuel Clemens, better known as Mark Twain - the author of *The Adventures of Tom Sawyer,* lived in Hannibal during his youth. He moved there with his family when he was four years old and left Missouri when he was eighteen to travel the world. Much of the area is a reflection of his many writings and the characters he brought to life. We stayed in Hannibal for three days waiting for rain to stop so we could cross into Illinois, but we only skimmed the surface of the cultural attractions to be experienced there.

One evening, after a long day on the road, we sat beside the Mississippi River in Hannibal. I was typing my website diary on my laptop. We were waiting, hoping to see some tugboats pushing their load of barges down the river. It truly amazed me how they could shove this string of what looked like boxcars (and could have been as far as I know) ahead of them and guide them exactly where they needed them to go. I always envisioned a tugboat pulling barges, not shoving them.

Our parking place was right next to a railroad track and as we waited, we heard the rumble of a train moving by. It was moving slowly, but the sight which grabbed our attention was two boys, maybe eight or ten years old, across the tracks from us. As the train moved between us, we could see the boys pick up rocks about the size of baseballs and place them on the track in front of the steel wheels. They would hold them on the track until the wheel was within inches of the stone, then step back and watch as the weight of this iron snake smashed the rock. My anxiety was soaring; my imagination was in full gear, but it was impossible to attract their attention over the chugging and clanging of the slow moving giant. We were spellbound by the possible disaster until the caboose finally passed by and we saw the two risk-taking buddies walking to their bikes on the hill next to the sidewalk. I could only think, "How many times in your life has God taken care of you when you did something really stupid?" I won't even try to count.

We crossed the Mississippi into Illinois on May 20, another milestone on this journey. We had only walked a few miles when a freshly washed, shiny new pick-up truck stopped by. The middle-aged man at the wheel put his head out the window and asked, "Is that your car back there along the road?" "Yes," we replied. "Do you need help?" "No, we are walking for the American Diabetes Association." With that this kindly man turned into a sneering brute; as he squealed off he shouted, "Great trick." I felt slapped! I wanted to cry. To think that someone saw us as two old people who had developed another scam for taking money from the naive made me sick to my stomach.

The man's reaction triggered a flashback to when we were in Oklahoma and called by a reporter from Oklahoma City. He questioned every aspect of our journey. Since I had called him previously to let him know what we were doing, he was suspicious. He couldn't understand why someone would actually walk across Mid-America without an ulterior motive. He didn't believe that our primary goal was to encourage others to challenge the road ahead of them, dream for what may appear to be lost because of disease or injury, make new goals, and acquire new dreams. We continued to suggest, "Today make a plan and tomorrow experience an adventure." His insults included the implication that we were only looking for limelight and insinuated that the only reason we were walking for the diabetes association was to receive favor from unsuspecting strangers.

We even had friends suggest that perhaps we didn't really walk the full 1038 miles. Since we had taken our car with us and returned to it after each couple of miles, their hint was, "who would know if you drove more and walked less?" We also had some who implied, since our fundraising was not nearly what we had hoped, maybe we kept some for ourselves and didn't forward it all to The American Diabetes Association. All the comments were very intimidating. Some of these people were bullies, some were caring friends, and some were just unknowing. If we had succumbed to our tumultuous inner feelings, if we had become obsessed with what others might think, we would never have experienced the greatest adventure of our lives. Helen Keller was once quoted as saying, *"Life is either a daring adventure, or it is nothing."*

Far too often, we let what one or two people say discourage us. Just think about it; what do you remember longest, someone saying something nice about you or if they say something bad about you? What does it take to stop you from reaching for your dream? Don't let a bully or an unknowing friend determine your destiny! They may only be trying to survive their own life. Find someone who believes in your dream, who will encourage you, and give your dream all you have. Life is about living, let's make it an adventure.

Except for the young Jay, this chapter focused mainly on people who could have destroyed our dream and caused us to cancel our journey for fear of "what would people think?" Do not fear people. Be afraid of that feeling that can rob you of your potential. Do you understand? Just one Jay makes up for those intimidating remarks and we met many "Jays" along the way. You will too!

Chapter 13
Fear, Friend or Foe?

It is my opinion that, the only time fear is an asset is when you are being chased by a bear.

But, you might say, fear sometimes causes people to make good adjustments in their health care. How many times have you seen someone who's had open heart surgery make a drastic change in their diet, add supplements suggested by their doctor, increase their amount of exercise and even quit smoking, drinking or whatever they believe might have been a contributing factor? Do they continue these changes the rest of their life? Why not? Out of fear, they made radical changes but, once they begin to feel better, the mental picture of all they went through dims and the fear subsides. So their commitment to change loses strength. The surgery may have opened the clogged arteries, but it did nothing to change what caused them to clog originally. Your desire for a full life must be stronger than the luring call of the culprits that brought about the problem.

Fear, or fright, is a temporary emotion which normally subsides once the immediate danger is removed. Fear should be replaced with knowledge and commitment. If the emotional fear remains, it not only causes stress in your body which can cause disease, but it also puts chains on your productivity. It will stop you from going forward into the unknown. Fear of failure is one of the most "crippling diseases" in our country today. To go forward into the unknown requires both wisdom and faith. It is important to look at the options, the costs, the possible problems, and make wise decisions about them. Then put your faith in the God who cares for you and guides your every step; trust Him. *"...I am the God of Abraham thy father: fear not, for I am with thee...."* (Gen 26:24)

Please allow me to share another type of fear, which is a temporary emotion but reoccurs again and again. Each recurrence sets the stage for immobilization in any given circumstance. I have a granddaughter, EmberLi Riner, who is a senior in high school. In most areas, EmberLi is one of the bravest persons I have ever met. One of her first solo driving experiences, after receiving her driver's license, was into downtown Dallas. Now, that requires courage! Even as a small child, when faced with a challenge, she would just straighten her shoulders, draw her cheeks in between her teeth and strut straight toward any obstacle in her way. (Sometimes that was this grandmother.) She never sees an object or situation too big for her to handle ... that is until she met the great, insurmountable "spider." It doesn't matter how small the animal is, she turns white under her salon-tanned complexion and, if possible, would become the invisible woman. I know this fear of spiders isn't uncommon. I also know it isn't easy to overcome, but it can be done. I challenge EmberLi, and anyone else who may struggle with the same type of fear, to take whatever steps are necessary to replace this fear with knowledge. After all, EmberLi, you might not have to wait four hours to get down the mountain to use a spider-free restroom if you just understood who you are!

> *And God said, 'Let us make man in our image, after our likeness: and let them have dominion over the fish of the sea, and over the fowl of the air, and over the cattle, and over all the earth, and over every creeping thing that creepeth upon the earth.' (Gen 1:26)*

That means that you should NOT be afraid of those spiders; if anything, they should be afraid of you. (They probably are.)

I know it's hard to believe, but it has been my observation that many people are afraid of getting well. Since our return to health in 2001, Ron and I have committed our lives to encouraging others to become an active participant in regaining and maintaining their health. Some people have a fear of loosing their disability insurance.

Their cry is, "But what if I get well for awhile and then it comes back again? Do you realize how hard it is to get on disability insurance?" No, I haven't done that, so I really don't know, but my reply is, "But what if you get well enough to lose your disability benefits and then it doesn't come back?" As I said earlier, only you can count the costs (and it's not all about the pocketbook) and decide how much you are willing to risk. How much is your health really worth to you?

(I pray that you will hear my heart before you cut off my fingers and toes for writing this paragraph.) While we were on our walk through the Midwest, in two different states we came upon rallies raising funds for cancer research. Each of them had a survivors' march or celebration; I'm not sure what they called it. When I saw the first one, I was very troubled in my spirit and mentioned it to Ron. I even asked him why I should feel so despondent because they were honoring survivors in such an ecstatic way. I knew if one of them was my loved one, I would also be overjoyed if they had survived cancer. In the next state where a rally was being held, we even walked in it for a few miles. But again, I grieved when the survivors took the track. What was wrong with me?

Since that time, and much soul searching, I have come to understand my emotional turmoil. I looked up the word "survive" in the dictionary and found it means "to live beyond the death of someone else or to outlive or outlast." I understand that, in the interpretation of the program, it means to outlast cancer. In no way does it belittle someone who died of cancer. But that still didn't comfort me. I finally discovered my answer. The word that fits these courageous individuals is not survivor. To me, the word "survivor" represents a passive stance. We can survive an earthquake by doing nothing other than, by chance, not being in a place where a huge boulder falls on us. The phrase that best fits these brave warriors is "overcomers." The definition of "overcome" is "to get the best of in a conflict or battle, or to defeat or conquer." This is a word of action! Every day of life should be more than surviving; it should be about being an overcomer. None of us knows if we have a tomorrow, but today we have a life to live. Those taking the track were overcomers and, yes, every day of life justifies a standing ovation!

I recently received an email with one of those messages that asks you to forward it to all of your friends. You know the kind I am referring to. This one, I felt, fit right into this issue of fear. The story went:

A sick man turned to his doctor, as he was preparing to leave the examination room and said, "Doctor, I am afraid to die. Tell me what lies on the other side." Very quietly, the doctor said, "I don't know." "You don't know? You, a Christian man, do not know what is on the other side?"

The doctor was holding the handle of the door; on the other side came a sound of scratching and whining, and as he opened the door, a dog sprang into the room and leaped on him with an eager show of gladness.

Turning to the patient the doctor said, "Did you notice my dog? He's never been in this room before. He didn't know what was inside. He knew nothing except that his master was here, and when the door opened, he sprang in without fear. I know little of what is on the other side of death, but I do know one thing, I know my Master is there and that is enough."

Author Unknown

To overcome fear, we must first identify it. Often it will appear as stress and/or anxiety. Sometimes we know what circumstances cause the stress, sometimes we don't. For example, we once owned a gasoline service station. After we had been there a few years, the EPA (Environmental Protection Agency) invoked some new laws regarding gasoline tank maintenance and ground control. Instantly, we inherited the liability for every person who held title to that property before us. In trying to meet the EPA standards and doing all that we could afford, and some that we couldn't, we found ourselves defaulting on payments. Talk about stress and anxiety! It looked like bankruptcy was inevitable. We were not incorporated, so what we had to lose was our home, (in Indiana our home would not have been protected in bankruptcy) plus the business, and our only source of income.

I lived for several months in literal panic. I would figure the budget for hours, trying to find money that wasn't there. One day, I decided I couldn't take anymore worry. I sat down and wrote a list of what were the absolute worst things that could happen because of this situation. The number one thing was, "What if the bank foreclosed?" I asked myself why that would be so bad because, by this time, I could think of nothing better than getting out of that situation. Guess what my answer was. Pride! All of our married lives, Ron and I had lived in that little town of 900 people where everyone knew everyone and we had worked hard to create credibility. What would they think of us now?

Number two was, "What if we lost our home?" It was an earth home with a picturesque view overlooking a small lake called "L Lake" (because of its shape). We had spent hours and months physically building that home. O.K., what would it mean if we were to lose it? Well, I didn't have the answer, but I wrote some of the things I did know. With families and friends, we knew that we would neither go cold nor hungry. If we lost the equity in our home, it wasn't all bad because we had lived in it for several years for not much more than rent would have been. And we had so many great memories. Memories like when our granddaughter, Alaina Martin, came for a visit. Shortly after her arrival, she always wanted to ride "Li'l Fella." Li'l Fella was a horse named in contradiction to his height, not for the lack of it. One time in particular, Alaina was still quite small, so I was leading the horse and walking on one side. Her mother, Kathleen, was walking on the other side. Alaina was feeling quite safe and secure, so she raised her hand to wave at cows in a near-by field. When she did this, she slid gracefully off the side of the horse and neither Kathleen nor I caught her. Li'l Fellow, being in mid-stride, stepped on her arm. We decided that it might be good to have an x-ray taken. At the emergency room, we tried to console Alaina, telling her they were just going to take a picture of her arm. But by that time, fear had overtaken her. I think the sobbing had more to do with her fear of the unknown than with the pain in her arm. Fortunately, there was no break and Alaina never decided to quit riding.

Another memory involved my niece, Tammy Koenig. She was learning to row a boat, and ended up deftly sliding her boat between a fisherman in his john boat and his bobber while I was rolling on the ground in laughter. Now that requires skill! Many, many such memories are planted in our minds. Such happiness and joy was found in that house, that I would always be thankful for it being a part of our past.

With the abilities we each had, I had no doubt that either of us would have trouble acquiring another job. So, I asked myself, "What is all this uproar about?" You guessed it! Again the answer was, "Pride!" Now, let me tell you a little about pride. According to the dictionary, the definition of pride includes "an excessive sense of one's own superiority." Once again, the old adage about pride going before a fall is found in the scriptures (Proverbs 16:18). Armed with this information, I finally understood that I had "nothing to fear but fear itself." (We've heard that many times, right?) If all I had to lose was pride, then it couldn't happen quickly enough. We finally submitted the problem to the Lord for His direction.

How did it all end? We were able to make an arrangement with the bank to sell the building and cancel our debt with them. We didn't have to file bankruptcy and Ron was able to move his mechanical repair business into a building on our home property. The fairy tale ending would be that we lived happily ever after. BUT, of course realistically life isn't that easy, we will always find another trial or fear lurking at the door. Nevertheless, I have learned that the quickest way for me to become an overcomer is to confront the issues and list the options. Then, I can make wise decisions. If fear creeps into life, identify it, analyze it, and let it motivate you to take a levelheaded stride toward peace and success. Fear is all about you. So think outside of yourself. Look for opportunities and let hope be your motivator.

Most everyone has seen or heard the "Serenity Prayer;" Lord, give me the strength to change what I can, the acceptance of what I can't and the wisdom to know the difference. My youngest granddaughter Savanna Riner gave me a lesson in dealing with what can't be changed when she was only three. I don't even remember what had occurred that devastated her, but she was crying uncontrollably.

After a few minutes of distress, Savanna saw that the outcome was not changing. She doubled up her little fists, rubbed them intensely across her tear-filled eyes, pasted a smile on her face, and stated, "I'm happy!" With that, she straightened her shoulders and bounced off to play. If there is an impossible, unmovable boulder in your path, move your path!

Chapter 14
Illinois Footprints

On May 20, 2004, we packed everything in our car once again and moved it to our starting point for the day. Tonight, we would be staying in Illinois. This morning, we were just a couple of miles west of the Mississippi River in Hannibal, Missouri. The heat of the day had already turned the air into steam as we approached the river. One of the disappointing points of the trip was that we were unable to walk across the river; the bridge had no place for pedestrians. That meant clocking the mileage on the car odometer as we crossed, moving the car that much further down the road on the far side of the river, walking back to the overpass and then returning to our vehicle. Thus, we made up for the miles that we drove across the Mighty Mississippi.

The day was hot as we continued our walk north on Highway 57. My journal entry for that day was:

O.K., you can call me Shaq. For those of you who don't know, Shaq is a basketball player with the L.A. Lakers. Why call me Shaq? Well, if you have watched him during a game you've seen how the perspiration drips off his face by the buckets. Today by 11:30 a.m. I had dripped enough I was wondering how long I would be able to endure...

As we walked past the farms and through an area that contained abandoned coal mines that had since been made into underground storage, it was a very real temptation to set up camp across from their entrances and bask in the cool, refreshing air spewing from those dark openings. However, not giving in to those urges, we walked through the industrial area and into Quincy, Illinois, where we collapsed in the Diamond Motel.

Joe and Maria Hildebrand, owners of the motel, pampered us, making our stay very affordable. They even taped the evening TV news segment of our walk, filmed just before we crossed the river, and presented us a copy of the video for our memoirs. The Diamond Motel is on the east side of Quincy along Highway 24. Arriving there was like a shot of energy. "24" would take us all the way into Logansport, Indiana, just thirty miles short of our final destination.

Remember that we had been in Hannibal, Missouri for three days waiting for the rain to subside. Do you know what happens to that water once the ground is full of it? It evaporates to become excessive humidity. By the second day in Illinois, I cut off my sweat pants and made shorts in anticipation of the hot days ahead.

At four-thirty in the afternoon that day, we were met by a photographer from the Quincy Herald-Whig. We had done an interview earlier by phone. I dreaded seeing that article in the paper! The day had been hot, humid, and windy. I could feel the grit over every exposed surface of my body. The wind used a mixture of hairspray, grime and sweat to plaster my sun-bleached, gray hair to my weary head. When that article was published on May 22, I wasn't a bit surprised. Ron looked as fresh as he did when we left the motel, and he always seemed to feel that way, too. But, there I was with my nature created coiffure. What can't be seen though is the reason for my tightly stretched shirt. Between the blouse and my boiling body, I had packed a water-soaked towel to help me tolerate the heat and the unrelenting humidity.

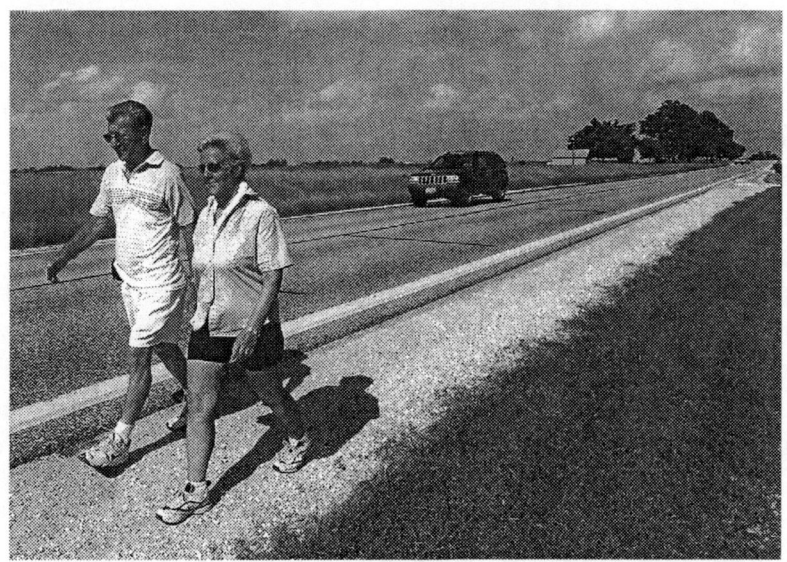

Walking east on Highway 24 near Quincy, Illinois. See that wet towel stuffed inside my shirt? Sometimes you'll do anything to try to be cool. (Photo by Philip Carlson, compliments of the Quincy [IL] Herald-Whig.)

Monday morning, May 24, found us back on "24" heading east through farmland. It was nearing noon and, as we were moving our car forward, we stopped in a small town called Camp Point. The restrooms at the local service station were beckoning. As we stepped from the car, we were met by Tammy. She asked if we would like to have lunch with them. "Well, um, now let me see." Our hesitation lasted about .5 of a second. The menu included turkey and dressing, green beans, etc., with a choice of salad and dessert. We were hosted by Camp Point's "Timber Point Healthcare" nursing home. They had seen Saturday's article in the paper and were watching for us to arrive in their area.

Tammy offered her office for us to have a quiet lunch, but we chose to join the residents. We sat with Effie and Alice. Effie was a little quiet, but possibly it was because she sat across from Alice. Alice and I chatted non-stop. It just happened that Alice had been a nurse for many years and had actually worked in this nursing home a few years before becoming a resident. Before we left, the staff blessed us with a contribution to the

American Diabetes Association and autographed the hood of our trusty, red sedan. Alice wanted to make sure her autograph noted her age of 92 years young. Ron and I both left hoping, if we ever need a nursing care facility, it would be as warmhearted as Timber Point Healthcare.

As I researched some of the Illinois information, I was reminded that Illinois is known as the Land of Lincoln. I discovered also that the state animal is the white-tailed deer and the state bird is the cardinal. That was information I already knew, or at least surmised, but do you know what really impressed me? Their snack food choice is after my own heart ... popcorn! As a matter of fact, I think I will take a break from my typing right now and pop a snack.

O.K., now I'm back on the road again. The next day, after leaving Camp Point, we were walking past flooded fields of farmland. Late in the afternoon, we were headed back to the car to call it a day, when I observed quite a commotion in the nearby fence row. Two blackbirds were flying near some shrubs and, from all the noise, I knew there was a bunch of hungry youngsters. I had to see!

Ron didn't care to see a nest of baby birds, but I headed out anyway. Let me tell you in advance that curiosity, combined with stupidity, can lead to trouble. I walked over to where the birds were. Between me and the nest, which I could see in the overgrown fence row, was a side ditch overflowing with water. I was able to jump it without a problem. Then I waded through knee-high grass until I reached the nest.

The leaves were thick and I peaked through the foliage into the blackbird home. I could see the dark markings on the naked, shiny body. By now, the kid in me had taken over and I wanted a closer look. The nest was about chin high, so I inched in closer, took my hand and pushed the leaves away just about an inch above that baby ... being sure not to touch it so the parent birds would not abandon it. Well, you may have already guessed, but the picture I got was not exactly what I was hoping for. When I saw that shiny skin start to uncoil, I realized that

I was not interrupting the dinner of baby birds, but disturbing the banquet of a snake.

Having grown up in farm country, I'm not much afraid of snakes, but neither do I like to be surprised by them. At that moment, Mother and Daddy Bird were on their own; they had no support from me. The situation was so disgusting that I no longer had the desire to see if there were actually any birds in the nest. I hoped that the gourmet meal only consisted of eggs. Where in the world is a gun when you think you want to use it?

Chapter 15
The Joy of Leaving Illinois

Illinois was certainly an adventure for us. We found that the people there were a little more trusting than in other states. They were certainly more comfortable donating to people walking along the highway for the American Diabetes Association. And they seemed more comfortable with giving their hospitality.

The Friday before Memorial Day, we left the Green Gables Motel in Rushville where the owner, Ron Sheppard, had gifted us with one of our nights' stay. After finishing our twelve miles for the day, we drove up Highway 24 to Peoria. We wanted to check on motels and the route we should travel through the city. We found that route 24 would take us through the industrial section and would go miles without a place to park the car, or go to the restroom, without getting off the main route. So, we turned to plan B. We had walked to Lewistown (southwest of Peoria on Highway 24) today, so we drove back through Lewistown to the Highway 136 intersection. Our alternate route would walk east on 136 and then north on 45 where we would again connect with 24. Saturday night, we would stay in Havana on Highway 136.

Saturday, May 29, 2004, my diary read:

O.K. Promise you won't laugh or make fun! Last evening after we came here to Havana and made our reservations for the next day we went out on the road and marked where we would be starting since we had changed our route [backtracking] ... now walking on route 136 rather than 24. Then today we went to our start point and walked forward another six miles. Something just didn't seem right! I always want to know which direction I am going, even though I can get my directions confused pretty easily. However, today seemed that we were walking south, not east. I kept trying to straighten it out in my mind, but it just persisted that we were headed south. Finally we started looking for a sign and sure enough we were headed south on 97 not east on 136. I am really disappointed with the Illinois road sign system. Wouldn't you think they would have put up a sign that said, "Hey, Dummy, you are going the wrong direction?" Now, before you ask, no, no, no we did not walk back to Havana! We just packed up our eight miles, drove back to Havana and then drove eight miles east on 136. We ended walking a little over 15 miles, giving us a total of 90.2 for the week and an overall total of 776.9 ... approximately 223 miles to go."

Ninety miles in one week, and an average of 15 miles per day for the week, set a record for our journey. One good thing came about because of our error in direction. If we had been on the right track, we would never have met the young lady who stopped to offer assistance. After hearing our story, she came back a little while later with a couple of bottles of nice, cold water.

Several times during our travels, we found ourselves without cell phone or Internet service; sometimes it would leave us three or four days at a time. It would seem a long time without communication to our family or friends. Surprisingly, no one appeared concerned when we didn't call. It reminded me of when I was little and my brother Larry and I would go away for hours at a time. I think that everyone thought, if something of importance happened, there would at least be one of us who would be able to relay the news.

I found that I am not the only curious person in the U.S.A. A couple of days later, we had just completed another 13 miles on highway 136 when a young man named Jeff stopped and asked if we needed anything. We discovered he had driven by us the day before. Then earlier in the day, he had driven by us again. He had copied our www.1000miles100days.com website address from our car's bumper and went home to find out just what was going on. However, he miscopied it as 100miles, not 1000miles, and couldn't find it. After giving us this much attention, he decided to drive by one more time and find out direct from "the horse's mouth." But he didn't just ask us about our trip, he invited us to his home for something cold to drink and to meet his wife Angela. He told us she was expecting us. We went back to our car, called it a day for walking, and followed him to his home in Fisher, which was only a couple of miles away. What a nice family and what a great way to end the day!

As we walked further east toward Rantoul, we noticed a two-story house. A ladder leaned against the side wall and about midway up the steep, second-story roof, shingles were standing up from a previous wind storm. Ron and I commented about how we would just call someone else to tackle that job. Even in our younger years, neither of us would have taken that kind of risk. When we approached the front of the house, we saw two men sitting on the front porch. We laughed and whispered, "Yep, that's exactly what we would do." We waved to the men and walked on. It was a very hot Saturday in early June and, as we passed by the men on the porch, we could see a wooded area about a quarter of a mile further up the road. We trudged on and found the roadside was well manicured, giving us an ideal spot to take a break in the shade of large overhanging tree branches. Reluctantly, we started back into the afternoon sun, headed for our car and its welcoming air conditioning.

When we got back to the house with the damaged shingles, we found Harold still relaxed on the porch swing and Jay propped against the railing. As we got near, Jay called out to ask if we would like something to drink. Ron asked if they had water. Harold replied, "We have lemonade." Harold opened the cooler and we gazed at the "refreshments" left from their fishing trip the day before. We decided to stick with lemonade. The only way we could partake of the other stuff, was if we were going to help fix the roof and needed some unwise courage, or pain killer in case of a fall. We were rested and refreshed, when an older model Camaro drove into the graveled driveway and seven or eight, men, women, and children scrambled out. It seems they were friends of Jay or Harold and had stopped to catch a couple of unsuspecting chickens feeding in the yard. Sunday dinner was about to be bagged, so it was time for us to return to the highway.

That evening, we drove to my brother's house in Parke County, Indiana. We were substantially ahead of schedule and even though his home was one and one-half hours away, it was well worth the extra drive. We were excited to be with family again, not to mention getting away from motels and fast food.

As children, it was always an exciting day for the family when my mother and father packed up hot dogs, chips and fixings and went to the woods. We would build a campfire and roast our wieners and marshmallows on sticks cut from one of the nearby trees. Larry and Caren have the ideal place and are always gracious in duplicating this family tradition.

The following Sunday morning, we attended church with them at the Linebarger Chapel United Methodist Church near Hillsdale, Indiana. Pastor Myers spoke about how we try to understand God; how we attempt to put an infinite God into our finite mind. He said that we make an effort to put God into a box. But God, of course, is bigger than our minuscule container. After the service we went for lunch at Turkey Run State Park with several of the church families. The park is quite close to the church.

The outing brought back memories of my Girl Scout leadership years. I remembered when I went walking with my girls on one of Turkey Run's trails at near dusk. Unfortunately, we under-estimated the amount of time to return back to the bridge near our camping spot and got lost in the woods. The woods were very dark, and we would occasionally come to a chained area with a sign stating, "Danger, Do Not Go Beyond This Point." We really didn't want to sleep under the stars, but we didn't want to chance someone falling into the ravine either. We found ourselves huddled together in a clearing where we could hear the camp sounds across a water-filled ravine, but could not find the bridge to get back. We spent the first portion of our night whispering, "One, two, three" followed by a synchronized scream of, "Help!" Finally, our call was answered by a male voice from the camp below us who said he would come after us ... to stay put. He knew exactly where we were. Relieved? Not quite. We weren't sure if we should hide or be glad he was coming. Was the voice from some kind of a pervert or a guardian angel? During the next half hour, my co-leader Linda Swartz and I rehearsed everything we knew about self-defense with our tribe. It turned out that our rescuer was a college student working that summer as a forest ranger. He was a red-headed guardian angel and a major attraction for my teen-age girls. Yes, adventure is a part of life.

O.K., that's enough reminiscing. Upon returning from our lunch with the church family, my sister Carol, and my brother Bruce, with his daughter Rachel, joined us for the infamous wiener roast that Larry and Caren expanded on. We sat in the cool evening air, hypnotized by the flickering flames, hearing the drone of the melodious insects, the call of the owl and whip-poor-will, and watching a raccoon in the trees. Enjoying this family moment, surrounded by the wonders of God's creation, only emphasized the morning's message: God is truly larger than any box and greater than any mind can conceive.

Early Monday morning we drove back to our marker, located west of Rantoul, and resumed our adventure. Just one week later, on June 12, 2004, about noon, we officially walked across the state line into Indiana. The event was a little disappointing. Highway 24 in Indiana was under construction; if there ever had been a "Welcome to Indiana" sign, it wasn't visible on this day. The only announcement was a sign saying we were "Leaving Illinois." Even without a welcoming sign, we really had a feeling of accomplishment and joy at finally reaching the fifth and last state of our journey.

Chapter 16
Russian Roulette Anyone?

Following an "early detection" routine is extremely important for a well managed healthcare schedule. Cancers, heart disease, even diabetes can be better managed if discovered in their early stages. So is early detection important? Yes! Dangerous? Yes! Relying on early detection as your main health management criteria is equivalent to playing Russian Roulette, only with a greater "chance" of lethal results. I'm sure you've heard of this deadly "game." You begin with a revolver holding six bullets. First, you remove all six bullets and re-insert only one. Now, you spin the chamber and put the barrel to your temple. Are you foolish enough to pull the trigger? Of course not! You have a one-in-six chance of losing your life with one reflex jerk of the trigger finger.

Now let me ask you, "Why not give your health care the same respect?" Current statistics show that one-in-two men will suffer from heart disease and one-in-three women will battle cancer. Would you be comfortable with putting say, two bullets in the gun? And let's say that you don't put the barrel to your head but to your chest. If you're lucky, a shot may only injure you, maybe you can be repaired. How good do you feel about those chances? Since statistics show that at least one-in-three will suffer from one of those two major diseases, what are your chances of escaping without at least one of hundreds of chronic diseases, if you don't take serious precautions? I could suggest that there is one-in-ten who survives life without a chronic disease, and I believe I would be estimating generously. However, I would also suggest in most cases, "that one" has contributed, by lifestyle, to that distinction.

Scientific research has suggested that 70% of ALL diseases are diet related. Research has also identified the necessity of glyconutrients (monosaccharides), essential fatty acids, and essential amino acids plus vitamins and minerals for healthy cells. Since our bodies are made up of organs, our organs made of tissues, and tissues consist of cells, how are we to have healthy bodies without healthy cells?

Let's go back to early detection. If you go to the doctor today for an "early detection" check-up, today may not be the day for that big bullet to fire. But you still have a nine-in-ten lifetime chance of receiving news that you have a chronic, if not deadly, disease if you do not become serious about maintaining a healthy lifestyle. A healthy lifestyle requires eating properly, using food supplements to provide necessary ingredients that are missing in our diets, exercising, and getting adequate rest.

I know this thought is very discouraging. I also know that a majority of you reading this book have probably already been diagnosed with a chronic situation. Chronic is defined as constant, unceasing, never-ending, or persistent. But let me encourage you by saying that there may be hope of lessening, if not reversing, those conditions without adding more drugs. When you switch to a healthy lifestyle management, you may not see the immediate results that you expect with medications. However, when you experience a decrease in symptoms, it will be because of increased physical condition, not a masking or cover-up of warning symptoms.

As we near the end of our story, I pray that you will understand that this journey was something we never thought would be a possibility for us. Even after we began our health management agenda, our hope was just to be able to function in a manner where we could enjoy watching our grandkids playing sports or be able to sit through a church service. In September 2001, Ron wasn't able to sit through an hour of church nor was he able to sit on bleachers at the sports fields more than a few minutes. If he sat outside in the cold (and in Texas, cold is not COLD) for a little while, we faced a real challenge for him just to get back to the car. There were occasions when I would have to drive us home after one of the grandkid's games, because he was unable to bend his legs enough to master the brakes and accelerator.

Our journey toward better health and this amazing trek started with the encouragement of a friend who, in our case, was my brother Dan. I'm praying that we may be the friend needed to encourage you. Your journey will start one step at a time. The first step is the decision to have a healthier life and who knows where the following steps will lead. We hope to make another walk similar to this one before our lifetime here is over. Every day, we are grateful for the ability God gave us through that first step.

Is the decision difficult? Are you afraid of failure? I think that eating properly scares everyone. What is "eating properly" anyhow? Does it mean giving up things that taste good? We have read that people should eat five to ten servings of raw, fresh fruits and vegetables per day. That's scary by itself. But the truth may be that five to ten servings will not be enough in today's American society because of the decline in nutrients found in our green-harvested, soil-depleted, and chemically-treated produce. There is an urgent need to supplement, to replace the glyconutrients, essential fatty acids, vitamins, and minerals that are often missing in our diet. That is where we started; then, we became more cautious and more educated about what we ate. We became more familiar with what supplements were needed to supply what we believed was missing in our diets. Once we began feeling better, we began exercising, too.

During our walk to Indiana, we spent more than eighty nights in motels. Our finances were very limited, so most of the time we ate in fast food restaurants. But every morning and every night, without fail, we swallowed our supplements and our health remained strong through the full 2,500,000 steps of our trek.

I recently read a book called *The Cost of Being Sick* written by Dr. Nicholas Webb. He talked about the benefits of prevention vs. treatment. The first benefit is preservation of your lifestyle. This was what we found when Ron was finally free of the arthritis that would have prohibited our adventure. As Dr Webb said, many in their retirement years are fighting for their lives, rather than living them.

Another benefit that also caught my attention was how prevention can also strengthen your finances. Let me suggest some figures to you. Dr. Webb wasn't talking about a $7.50 bottle of vitamins and minerals per month. The figure he used is $100.00. If a person started at the age of forty-five purchasing $100.00 per month of quality supplements, by the age of 65 he would have spent $24,000. Studies show that a couple retiring today at the age of 65 will need approximately $160,000 to cover their retirement medical expenses, if they are not covered under an employee health insurance plan. With the current rate of inflation, that figure is expected to rise to somewhere between $500,000 to $2,225,00 in the next 20 years. Dr. Webb noted that financial security and even avoiding bankruptcy during our senior years could depend upon a commitment to practice prevention rather than relying on "treatment only" for our health and wellbeing. There's a lot of difference between spending $24,000 or $500,000.

What is more important to you than investing $100.00 per month in your wellbeing? Could it be a frozen, chocolate-flavored coffee topped with whipped cream each day? Or maybe you stop for a couple of sodas daily. If you have a family, the amount for food supplements could zoom to four or five hundred dollars per month. Choosing to spend that amount on your health might mean that you don't trade cars as often or the house you buy may not be your dream home, but how important will those things be when you or a family member lands on one of those bullets that only one-in-ten may avoid? Playing Russian Roulette is stupid, even more so when only one chamber is empty!

I can hear already the groans of some of you reading this book. You may be saying, "That sounds great, but you don't understand. I'm not living in my dream home nor am I able to trade cars. If I drink soda or a flavored coffee, it is only on special occasions for a treat. If I take one-hundred dollars out of my income this month, my family won't eat." I want to encourage you. I'm not asking for the impossible. All I ask is to do the best you can. You can start by limiting sweets, sodas, and harmful fats from your diet and add more uncooked, fresh fruits and vegetables to your menus. Also make sure that you and your family get both adequate exercise and rest. These two things by themselves can improve your health and lessen your chances of being sick. In the end, you may find that $100.00 per month or more will be saved by your lack of medical needs. We did.

Please don't make the mistake that I did! I have wished many times that I had known and disciplined myself and my family to make the changes that I ask you to make. But, I didn't! By making better choices earlier, I may have been able to help them avoid the medical challenges that they have faced. Had I known and believed that I could make a difference, their lives may have been changed. No one can go back and change the past, but we can make a decision that, "from this moment forward I will do the best that I am able."

Russian Roulette is not a game! Your health is not a disposable commodity. It's a gift. God miraculously created our bodies to heal themselves if they are supplied with the right components. If you have good health, cherish it and protect it. Don't wait for your early detection exam to reveal a catastrophe. If your health is less than desirable, start now to rebuild from where you are today. Challenge that road ahead!

Chapter 17

Back Home Again in Indiana

As we near the end of our trip, I've only touched some of the highlights of our experiences. So let me give you a look at what our average day was like as we walked through Texas, Oklahoma, Missouri, and Illinois. We would usually get up around seven or seven-thirty, about two hours before we planned to begin walking. We would dress for the day, which included a good cover of sunscreen. Ron would go for breakfast and his two cups of coffee while I fixed my face and hair. Ron would bring me something to eat, which usually contained an apple and muffin if we were eating the continental breakfast at a motel. But, if there was no breakfast with our room, it would usually be a sausage biscuit sandwich and/or hash browns from a fast food restaurant. I would chow it down while he packed ice, food and supplies for the day. After swallowing our powder and capsule nutrient supplements, we would set out for the highway.

Sometimes our start location was as far as twenty-five or thirty miles from where we stayed, depending on how far affordable, livable motels were. Sometimes it was hard to find that combination and still stay within our budget, which made complimentary rooms a greater blessing. On the days we moved to a new location, we had to include an extra half-hour to pack and check out in the morning and guess at how long it would take to find another place in the evening.

If we were near a town, we could stop for lunch at a local eatery, but if not, we would eat from the supplies in our car. We carried things like apples, bananas, breakfast bars, crackers, and nuts. Plus, we always carried an ample supply of bread, peanut butter, and honey … and, yes, I still enjoy peanut butter and honey sandwiches.

During our afternoon stint, we would plan to be back at the car around four o'clock. That seemed about the time I was ready for a little time on my behind and an infilling of encouragement. An afternoon snack and a brief study from Rick Warren's *Purpose Driven Life* would provide the strength I needed to go again for another hour or two. As we studied from Warren's book, neither Ron nor I came up with how we would accomplish what we felt strongest we were meant to do. After our new lease on life, following what seemed to be at the end of our "best years," our drive was to encourage others to manage their "preventive" health care. We also wanted to be financially involved in building a church. I think many people are given an idea, a plan of action, of how to accomplish their goals. However, we haven't received a clear cut pattern.

When we conceived our dream of walking through the mid-states of our country, our thoughts were to convey to others struggling with health issues that there is hope, to create a life that goes a step beyond the average crowd, to raise money for the American Diabetes Association, and an adventure to share for our 50th wedding anniversary. There was no thought of using that experience to write a book; that thought came only after hearing from several people who read our diary on the www.1000miles100days.com website suggesting that I should write a book. They encouraged me with comments that said they thought I had the talent to write in a conversational, interesting manner. Just like the dream of the stroll to Indiana, a thought that couldn't be ignored was birthed. Yes, I thought, this was a way we could support others as they "Challenged Their Road Ahead." I hope that writing a book doesn't take skill; I don't know how to write a book. I trust that willingness and courage to follow that undeniable beckoning deep inside will suffice. If you are harboring a passion inside but feel incapable of completing the task, find someone who knows what you lack and let them help complete your "shortfall" areas; dare to seek and pilot your destiny.

Usually after our study in *The Purpose Driven Life*, we would walk a few more miles and determine by five or six o'clock in the evening to call it a day. However, one day we walked 18.1 miles, which was our personal record. On that day, we walked a little later after stopping for a McDonalds' hot fudge sundae. That was a rare treat though, because we knew that the instant surge of energy was due mostly to the sugar in the treat and would not maintain the endurance to accomplish our goals. But on this hot day, as we were trudging past those golden arches, our steps just kept turning toward the door … restroom break? Well, maybe, but that cool, refreshing treat was a powerful, underlying draw.

Our first day in Indiana was a hot and muggy one. We didn't get started on the road until almost 11:00 a.m. because of a morning rain. About an hour later, we walked across the state line and onto the road reconstruction of Indiana's stretch of U.S. Highway 24. As we walked along the narrow strip between the new blacktop and the flooded side ditch with its soggy grass, we saw hairless baby rabbits lying beside the freshly repaved roadway. We could not determine if they had drowned from the recent rain, or if their nest had been destroyed by road construction equipment. I always found it a little depressing to see animals that had died along the road, but we felt very blessed that we never found a human body. I can say that the thought of that possibility was one of my major concerns while traipsing the highways.

It was on a Saturday when we walked into Indiana. We followed "24" through Kentland and decided to spend the weekend with my sister Carol, near Claypool, Indiana. That was about 90 miles further than our stopping point for the day, so we left the highway early. The car was filled with our things after checking out of the motel that morning, so we could head to Peru where we met with Carol, my brother Bruce, and his daughter Rachel for dinner. From there, we drove on to Carol's house where we would stay until Monday morning. On Sunday, we went with Bruce to the *New Foundations Ministries* church, which met in a converted theater in Wabash. Pastor Rick Tolley spoke on "Possessing the Promises of God," using the sixth chapter of Joshua as the text for his message. In his introduction, he said: "The Bible we hold in our hand contains hundreds of promises to those who have given their entire life over to God." He went on to ask, "If [these promises] are ours, why are we unable to experience them in our lives?" His answer was that we have been unwilling to pay the price. We want the blessings and privileges without the responsibilities. He pointed out, "That which costs nothing means nothing." I admit I had to reflect on how little we seem to appreciate our freedoms in the USA, and what a great price has been paid for us to have those freedoms. Do we even grasp how grateful we should be? Would we be willing to pay the ultimate price to maintain these freedoms?

Bruce's wife Jackie and Carol provided so much great food for Sunday's meals that we went back to our walk on Monday feeling a little pudgy, but satisfied. They paid the price and we enjoyed the blessing. I'm sure that wasn't what Pastor Tolly was saying, but my mind went a few steps further ... *NOTHING* is free. Everything cost someone something, including the greatest gift ever, salvation from our sin.

Chapter 18
Wanted: Dead or Alive

Monday found us, on the road again in Indiana. We had enjoyed this journey, but were getting excited! In only a few more days we would reach our destination. I know everyone would not have found as much pleasure in this trip as we did, but my utmost desire is that everyone could find an adventure that would provide equal satisfaction in their lives. My greatest concern and compassion is to motivate and encourage those who have lost their lives to sickness, disease, or accident, but are not dead. I am not referring to those who may be in a coma or physically or mentally unable to make choices for their life, but I may be speaking to their caregivers. We frequently forget that, most often, the caregivers' lives are changed dramatically, and any normalcy of their life is lost.

A few years ago, someone asked if I could change one thing in my life, what would that be? I thought a little while and answered that I didn't think that I would make any changes. Of course, things have happened that I didn't like, I've done things that I regret, and I've made decisions that were definitely wrong. But, if I went back and changed even one of those things, I don't think I would be where I am today. Today, I have peace and joy; I don't know where another path may have led me. I hope I can encourage anyone who has lost his or her "life" because of circumstances beyond their control, to combine your hope with mine and discover joy and adventure in whatever situation you may be in.

When I am discouraged, I find joy and tranquility in contemplating God's creation. It is such a mystery to me. First, I begin to think, "how large is the mind of God to even imagine all that is around us, let alone speak it into being?" And when I think of speaking, I am utterly amazed at His creation of language. When He created us, we came with the tools for speaking. Have you considered what He had to provide before He could even give us that ability? Ears, mouth, tongue? Yes. But what we see on the outside is hardly what it takes to hear. Think of all the nerves and whatever else in the brain it takes to transmit those sound waves and turn them into identifiable words. But where did those sound waves come from? You might say that they come from our throat, our "voice box." But, "How did He decide what sounds would translate to 'tree' or 'cat'?" Even after He made that decision, how did He get them to travel a distance on what we call "sound waves" into the ear canal so that we can hear distinctive sounds that make words? And what in the world is a sound wave anyhow? How do you suppose it got there? Even Helen Keller, who could neither hear nor see, acquired the ability to communicate and, as I quoted earlier, said, "Life is either a daring adventure, or it is nothing." The questions are easy; I may never know the answers.

Another aspect that inspires my day is thinking about the living things on our planet. My family members, each with their own uniqueness, all the animals with their individual differences, and the plants created in so many forms, are all a fascination to me. Science has come a long way in figuring out some of God's mysteries, but with all our technology man cannot create a living thing. We have learned how to abstract cells from living plants and animals to grow bigger, better versions or even clones, but we cannot create a seed or a single cell. I mentioned my fascination with how God created language and, I want to remind you again, that there is also a type of language, a communication between and within our cells. With everything I learn and see, I never cease to be astounded!

Have you considered the furniture you're sitting on and the other pieces around you? Each piece came from a dream or vision of somebody. The design was first formulated in someone's mind. Each building, tower, auto, plane, coin, or landscape design was first conceived within a person's mind. What is a mind and where did it come from? How is it different from the brain? I'll let you explain that to me if you would like.

A few days ago, during my prayer time, I looked up at the ceiling fan in my bedroom. What I saw wasn't a surprise, because I have known for a while that it needed cleaning badly, but there were just some things I decided to let go until I completed this book. That ceiling fan was one of them. But what usually happens when I look at it didn't happen. Normally, I would feel a little down on myself because I don't like house cleaning, but I do like a clean house … kind of a Catch 22. But what happened on this day was different. I looked at all that dust stacked up on the blades, in some places even hanging from the edge about a half inch. I looked at the piles and began thinking about each particle of dust dangling there. Dust is so fine that a small puff of wind blows it away. So how did it get stacked up on a whirling device? I thought, "Since God created dust, he must have given it the ability to hold frantically as those blades hummed above my bed. How did He do that?"

I encourage you <u>not</u> to become a, "Why me, Lord?" person. Have you ever wondered why a child is always asking, "Why?" Maybe it's because he hasn't yet learned that the world is possibly <u>not</u> supposed to revolve around him. Let me stimulate your thoughts with some "why" questions. Why does a red-headed woodpecker go up the tree with his head up, while a nuthatch will come down the tree with its head down? I don't think you will see them in reversed positions. Why does your hair grow from the scalp, rather than from the ends of the hair? Did God already know that I would burn off the ends with my curling iron? Why can I walk on ground, but not on water? Was that just reserved for Jesus and Peter? And why does water get hard when it gets cold rather than when it gets hot? I know there is a scientific reason, but why? Why does the sun come up in the east instead of the west and why do European cars have steering wheels on the right side instead of the left? Is it so they can ride closer to the oncoming vehicles, since they drive on the left rather than on the right like we do? And why DO we drive on the right?

In revealing my "why" thoughts, my desire is to encourage you to think outside any consuming situation. Do not fixate on your circumstances. Anything that monopolizes your thoughts also controls you. Why not let your thoughts be fixated on or monopolized by a God who cares for you? Let Him and His goodness overwhelm you. Anger, and frustration is a form of anger, is one of the most consuming emotions we have, but it's difficult to live a life full of anger if we quit focusing on how we were wronged. If I determine to treat each person I meet today with the same respect that I would give Jesus himself, I believe I can "live life" by serving those around me. Maybe I can't do anything but give a smile. Or maybe I know someone who would like a phone call. When we start living to bring joy to others rather than looking for others, or things, to bring joy to us, we will no longer have to search for happiness, it will find us.

Since I have experienced, and seen in others, the results of how nutrition can change the quality of life, I want to share that information with those I see facing chronic health conditions. Many people I've met are resistant or skeptical. Sometimes they are just weary of trying various things; sometimes, they are still trying to come to grips with their situation and just want someone to cry with them. I think that is why God created each of us with unique personalities. As I mentioned before, Ron is one of those who feels your pain and despair; he is one who will cry with you. I'm cut from a different pattern. If I see a problem, I want it fixed just as quickly as possible, whether it is in your life or mine. What is your gift, your personality? How were you molded? It doesn't matter; there are those who need you. If you are walking through a life of chronic illness, you have an understanding of those experiencing a similar walk that I don't have. I haven't gone through that experience, but Ron has. What I'm suggesting, encouraging, is that you live to give to others. You have a purpose. We met some of you on our walk.

Chapter 19
The Last Leg

We left Kentland on June 14 and walked through several small towns along Highway 24. I felt rather melancholy as we strolled through Goodland, Remington, Wolcott, Reynolds, and into Monticello. I remembered my mother talking about these towns from her childhood days, as places she had visited or lived near. Many historical homes and quaint shops still remain along this route.

As we neared Monticello, it began to sprinkle and soon started to rain harder, so we returned to our car and drove into town to search for a motel. Monticello is a resort area near Lake Shafer with Indiana Beach nearby. By now, our funds were on their last leg. Motel rooms were more than we could afford, so we were seriously considering the Fishers' Bed and Breakfast in Rochester. Actually, the Fishers are Ron's brother Jim and his wife Mary. They don't really have a bed and breakfast, but many of their friends and family seem to think so, including Ron and me. We had just about given up on a motel room when we stopped at Best Western. When the manager heard our story, he put us up in a very nice room, free. I wish all those who helped us along the way, and after we arrived, had some way of feeling just how grateful we are for their help in making this journey possible. And by helping us, joined our effort to promote awareness of the diabetes epidemic and provide funding for research into treatment and cure.

On June 17, 2004, we walked through Monticello. The previous day we had reached the west edge of the city, after being slowed by a morning rain. When we were forced off the road, we went to Monticello's newspaper, *The Herald Journal*, and spoke with their reporter, Doug Howard. For the article he wrote, he photographed us tying our shoes ... getting ready for the end of the trail. We were now approximately 60 miles from our destination. Our minds were buzzing with thoughts about the finish line. If we walked our earlier goal of 10 miles per day, we would only have six days remaining. If we walked our daily average of 12.3 miles, then the end would be five days. And if we covered 15 miles a day, which was quite doable for us at this point, we would finish in four days. At this time our emotions were running high, but in opposite directions. "We are almost there and several days early. Let's hurry and see just how quickly we can do it." Or, "We are nearly at the end of this adventure. Do we really want it to end? Should we drag our feet to extend it a couple of days?"

We continued east on State Road 24 through Idaville, Burnettsville, and Lake Cicott. Ron continued finding his treasures along the roadside. This time it was a fishing rod and reel that must have fallen from someone's boat. Looking for different kinds of treasures, I found beautiful lilies and other early summer blooming plants that blossomed in Vel Benedict's garden. She graciously allowed me to photograph them. Some of the pictures I added to our website; some I enlarged and framed once we returned home. They hang on my wall as a reminder of the beauty of the people and the country we live in. As we got near Logansport, Ron found a wallet with the ID of an area high school student. Before the evening ended, we had called the phone number listed in the papers inside and returned the wallet to its owner. This was the second wallet that Ron found among roadside rocks and weeds. The first one was near Jefferson City, Missouri. That one he took to the police station. We never heard more about it, but the young man from Logansport sent a nice thank you note.

Now we had moved our belongings to Jim and Mary's "bed and breakfast" in Rochester. It was absolutely wonderful to finish the day and spend the evening with family and friends. Sometimes that would include Gene and Karen with their family or Virgil and Sue and their family. On Saturday, June 19, we met that cold front that I was concerned about back when I cut off my sweat pants. That morning the temperature was 59 degrees. Brrrrr. BUT, it was a good day for walking. The brisk temperature kept us moving just to keep warm and by evening we were six miles out of Rochester, only sixteen miles left. We could do that in one day! But, we decided to relax and use Monday and Tuesday to complete our journey.

Monday, we walked to the east edge of Rochester. That left only nine miles before reaching our destination. On Tuesday, June 22, 2004, we started a little later in the day and walked along S.R.14 toward Akron. We were visited frequently by friends who found us walking along on the narrow edge of the highway. We had been instructed not to enter Akron until five-thirty, but we weren't sure why that time was chosen. About mid-afternoon, when we got back to our car, we drove down one of the nearby country roads to find a grassy side-ditch. Without entering the town, it was the only place to relieve the pressing call of nature. We had only been back on the main street for a couple of miles when a friend stopped and asked, "Where were you? We came out and went all the way back to Athens and couldn't find you. Someone told us that they had seen you near Lake 16." Athens is a small community about half way between Rochester and Akron and Lake 16 lies between Athens and Akron. I think I just sort of mumbled through that answer.

What we couldn't know, see, or hear was the buzz we created in Akron. Ann Allen, the *Akron News* reporter for the *Rochester Sentinel,* had arrived and a WNDU TV, Channel 16 newscaster from South Bend, Indiana was waiting at the west edge of Akron for our arrival. Peg and Harvey Arthur, with their daughter Becky Gearhart, had posted a welcome sign for us and were there to take photos of us for the memorable occasion. Several friends and family were also there to greet us as we finally completed the last steps of our journey. Jim was taking pictures while Mary followed us into town driving our car. Our final steps were escorted by the City Police, fortunately as an honor.

The news reporters were asking questions like:

"Would you do it again?"

"Yes, in a moment's notice."

"How many pairs of shoes have you worn out?"

Both of us were still wearing our first pair of Nikes. However, I had purchased another pair and wore them a couple of days to break them in, "Just in case." Mine were looking pretty fragile.

"Did you ever think you would have to quit?"

Only once, when I stubbed my toe on a bed leg in the motel. I'm sure glad it didn't actually cause any damage to my toe … but it did hurt. I don't think anyone would have believed me if I told them that I wasn't going any further because I stubbed my toe in the room. Would you?

"Were you ever afraid?"

No. We didn't meet anyone who appeared to be a possible threat, no particularly aggressive dogs, and the serious storms were either at night or on Sunday when we weren't walking. We felt the prayers of friends and family and it seemed God had his umbrella over us the entire way.

"How much money were you able to raise for the American Diabetes Association?"

Only $456.25. That was a real disappointment to us. When we thought we would have drivers to go ahead of us and promote our fund raiser, we had high hopes of collecting $100 per day. That would have been nearly $10,000 but since we only met people along the highway, we found few who wanted to contribute.

"Being together 24/7 for nearly 100 days, did you find you raked on each others nerves and end up arguing a lot?"

No. We didn't argue once during that time. That was Ron's fault. He won't argue unless he is sure he's right, so I figured out a long time ago that it was rather fruitless arguing with someone who is right. This adventure actually drew us closer, having the same goal, doing the same things, and enjoying the same explorations.

"What next?"

We would like to do more walks, especially if we can get others to participate. We are considering such things as "wheel chair strolls" and trips for others who have limitations. We feel that our mission in life is encouraging others to do what THEY can do, not what we have done.

Ron's oldest brother Ralph had three children, Jane, Diane, and Ed. They were there, with their spouses and families, to welcome us home. Ralph is no longer alive, but his presence was felt in the company of his family. We're sure he would have been there with all his wise cracks (or should I have said, wisdom?). Ralph's kin treated us to dinner at *Sloane's Fine Food and Spirits,* where we were joined by Jim and Mary. Our spirits were different than those advertised and ours WERE fine.

Were we surprised to find the crowd and bustle at the west edge of Akron, Indiana, this small town of less than 1000 people? Well sort of, but some of our friends, checking on us while we were still back a few miles, were leaving hints. What a bitter sweet moment. We accomplished our goal and we were embraced by family and friends as they shared this moment with us. But – the trip was over. This adventure had ended. Mission accomplished! As the reporters asked, "What next?"

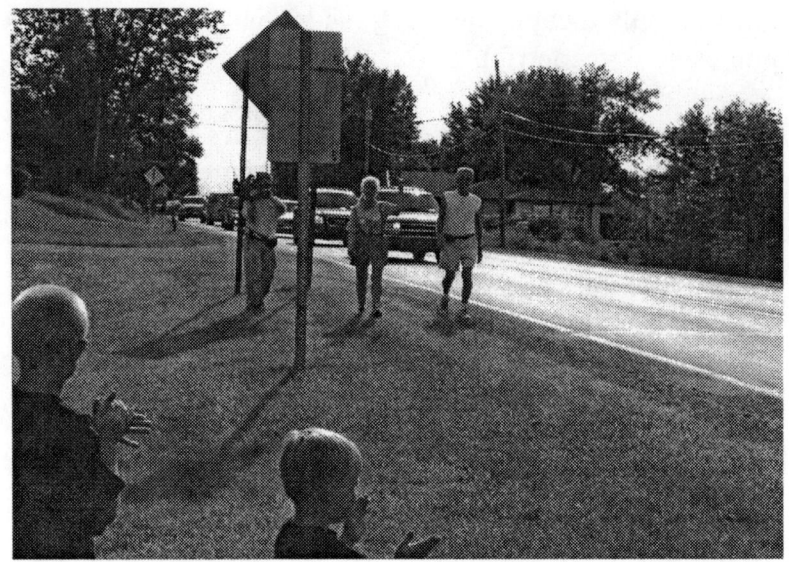

Akron, Indiana! We arrived, even ahead of schedule.

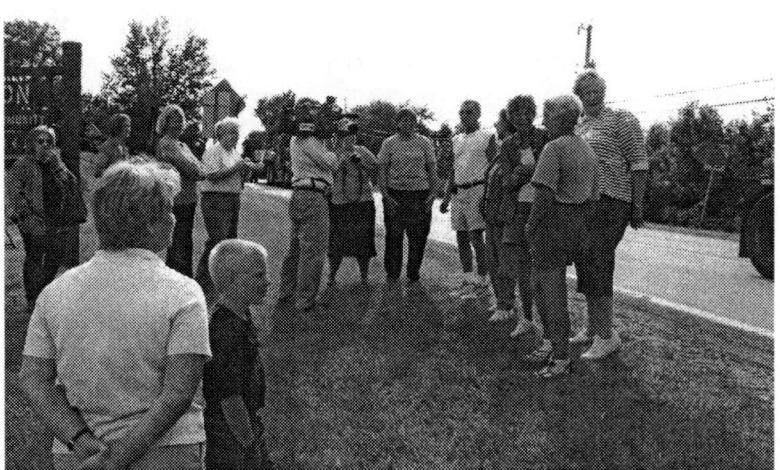

These reporters, friends, and family were some of those who welcomed us upon our completion of the 1038 miles, traveled on foot, to return "home" to celebrate our 50th wedding anniversary.

We had ten wonderful, relaxing days that we spent with family and friends before the 4th of July parade. It seems that every year the whole community, the whole country for that matter, goes to great lengths to help us celebrate our anniversary. Actually, the truth is that Akron was settled on July 4, 1836, and you know about the other July 4th ... the celebration is about their history, not ours.

Rick and Kathleen were unable to stay for our anniversary celebration, but they were in town for Kathleen's mother's birthday and had dinner with us. I am always amazed how Rick is able to keep people laughing, even while going through his own health challenges and discomforts. While we enjoyed these moments with Rick and Kathleen, Ron's family prepared our car for the next day's parade.

Saturday, July 3, 2004, found us in line for the town's birthday celebration parade. Usually, this event would have been held on the fourth but, since the holiday fell on Sunday this year, they chose Saturday instead. It was hot. Mary was there, dressed in her ice-padded vest, to drive our car and Jim was doing the photography. (Sorry, he forgot to open the lens on the camera.) We bought candy to throw to the spectators and Ron found a couple of children to toss it for us. What we didn't anticipate though was how fast the parade would move, and how many friends the kids would see to throw candy to. We realized pretty quickly that we had to carry the baskets and let them run to us for candy; otherwise, we probably would have found them at the end of the parade following the big Pike's trucks and equipment.

The only unexpected incident during our participation in this celebration was when Ron opened the trunk of the car to refill his candy supply. What he didn't realize was that he had stepped into the cords tied to the cans dragging behind the car in remembrance of our wedding day. It would have been a great scene for a movie. Even after 50 years of marriage, I didn't know Ron could dance like that! First hopping on one foot while trying to get the other one free, then trying to run up to the car with cans clanging along, trying to get enough slack to hop again in hopes of freeing his entangled foot. He breathed a deep sigh of relief when Mary finally saw his predicament and stopped the vehicle. Honestly, I was kind of enjoying his new challenge.

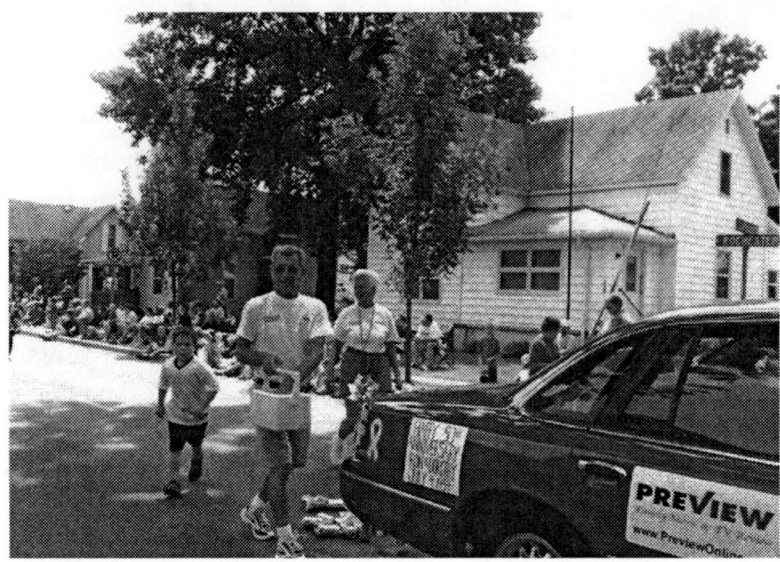

It works out great that Akron, Indiana celebrates the anniversaries of the founding of our country, the founding of Akron, and our wedding date on July 4 each year. This year, 2004, was an exception since the 4th fell on Sunday so the celebration was July 3. (However, the celebration wasn't really about us ... We just invited ourselves.)

On Sunday morning, July 4, 2004, we headed to the Pleasant Hill United Methodist Church. Pleasant Hill is a small country church located about halfway between the rural communities of Akron and Macy, near where I grew up. This was where we were married 50 years ago. We went early to hear the morning message by their pastor, Wayne Balmer. He spoke about what freedom really is, as we were preparing to renew our wedding vows. I think it was just coincidence, after all it was the 4th of July.

Immediately after the service, we were joined by 61 friends and family members to celebrate our special occasion. We felt very honored and humbled by their presence. However, as I turned around from speaking with a friend and checked to see where Ron had gone, I did a double-take. I wasn't sure I was seeing what I thought I saw ... the smiling face of the last person I expected to be there. This had been a well kept secret. Ron's brother Red lives in Bradenton, Florida. Red had been dealing with some very serious health problems and was constantly in our prayers ... that he would be able to go home from the hospital soon and then that he would be strong enough to remain at home. But here he was, sitting in the middle of the church with his grandson, Jay Young, who had flown with him. I cried. God had honored us by making this possible. Our joy was complete!

Brian and Krista and their children, Brant, EmberLi, Savanna, Caleb, and Roc, along with Savanna's friend Donnie were there to organize everything. What a great job they did, considering they didn't even arrive in Indiana until Saturday afternoon. They were not sure they could make the trip at all! Krista led us as we recognized each one of our immediate family members and spoke a little about them individually. Family is very dear to us and we believe that it was only by the support of our families that, what started as two troubled, teenage kids, survived 50 years of marriage.

My sister Kathy helped engineer the reception prior to our arrival, then Krista supervised as family and friends put it all together between the church service and our anniversary observance. We will be eternally grateful to each one of those who helped make the entire occasion, starting even before March 15 and ending long after July 4, an adventure that will live in our memory the rest of our lives.

Brian and Krista are ordained ministers and Brian officiated as we renewed our vows. Then he led us in this prayer:

> *Today we cannot foresee the future any more than we could in 1954. But today, we stand before you again, promising to love and honor each other until that day that death may part us on earth, but knowing we will live together with you in eternity.*
>
> *Lord, we ask your blessing on the remainder of our earthly journey and we pray for your strength as our strength may grow dim. We pray for your peace in the trials we may face, and we pray your hand will be over our families as our hands may grow weak.*
>
> *Lord, we submit ourselves and our families to you for your purpose.*
>
> *In Jesus' name we pray, Amen.*

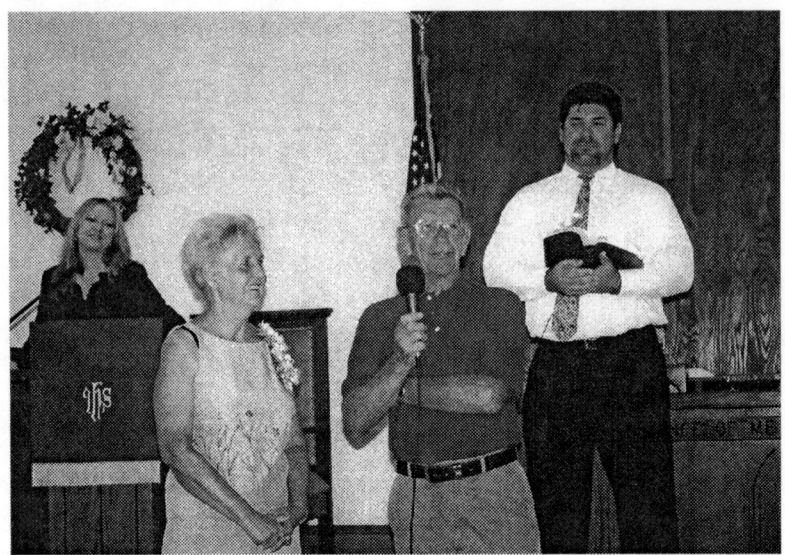

Sometimes Ron gets emotional and finds it is hard speaking about how much his family means to him. (Photo at Pleasant Hill Church just prior to the service for renewing our vows with Brian and Krista.)

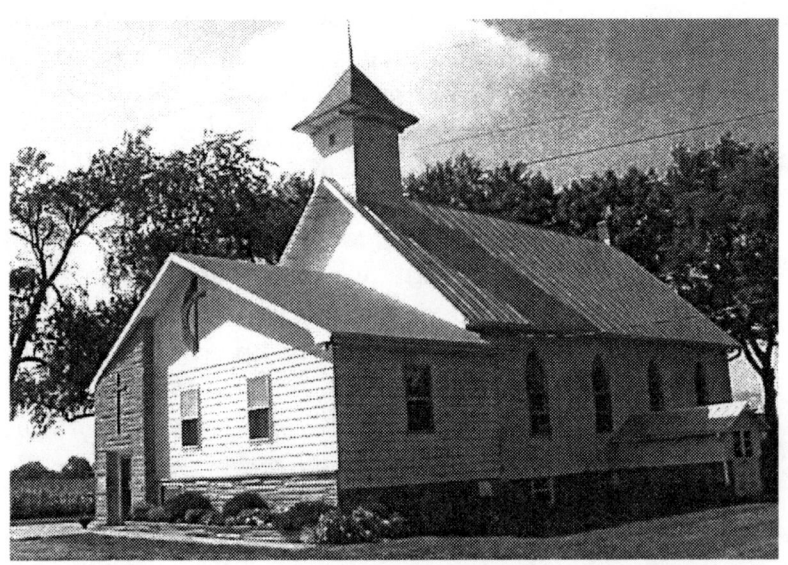

Pleasant Hill United Methodist Church, July 4, 2004.

Chapter 20
What is Your Story?

It has been my desire, through this book, to share the changes that took place in our lives, about what we did that brought them about and why we, at the age of 66 and 67, were able to walk 1038 miles from Dallas, Texas to Akron, Indiana. I wanted to share the experiences that we had along this journey and I also wanted to give you an insight into the homes where we grew up. I believe God created within us, even before we were born, a resilience which helped us choose a lot of right decisions. At the same time, He gave us the freedom to select wrong directions, too.

My story is about how we were able to turn back the hands of time on our aging conditions, how our childhood experiences affected our life's decisions, and how our beliefs empowered us to step out and attempt something, as far as we knew, no one else had ever done. That "something" was our anniversary stroll. However, that walk was only a stepping stone to what we believe God intends for us to do with our retirement years.

What is your story? How can it be used to help others? We believe that you have a message only you can give and that we, and uncounted others, can learn from your experiences. It is our prayer and our desire to motivate you, to encourage you, to help you determine your reason for living and make whatever changes you need to accomplish it. If you don't have a dream or a defined objective, I pray that our story inspires you to dare to dream and seek your purpose. I want to urge you to jump out into that great world of the unknown and find an avenue of impact into the life of someone else, whether it's only one person at a time or through mass media. You have a purpose and if you don't already know what that purpose is, I challenge you to search until you find it. It may be easier than you think!

Writing this book has been a struggle for me. First, I have been studying glyconutrients for the last three years, since we started taking them, and now I am enrolled in a nutritional course certified by The University of Miami School of Medicine. But in searching these dietary studies, I find the more I learn, the more there is to learn. I can only share what I have found and experienced and what I have observed in others.

During my first week of writing, I went to a conference where the speaker was a highly educated doctor in the field of nutrition. Even though she spoke about cell-to-cell communication, she never mentioned the eight monosaccharides or glycoproteins research has determined as necessary for proper cellular communication. Dr. Emil Mondoa writes in *Sugars That Heal*:

> *Saccharides enable cells to give and receive instructions, respond to each other's needs, know when to stop multiplying, and respect each other's space. Virtually every change within our multicellular bodies, from conception until death, is to some degree mediated by this language of sugars.*

Since these monosaccharides, or glyconutrients, were so instrumental in restoring a good quality of life for us, I couldn't imagine a seminar on nutrition without discussing them. But my question to myself was, "Why would anyone listen to me? I don't have any degrees." (Unless you want to count the GED I received at the age of fifty-eight, or my beautician's or realtor's licenses.) The only force that keeps me writing this is my strong belief that God has a message He wants me to write, that there is someone He wants to hear it. Could that be you, could it be my grandchildren? I don't know the answer, I'm just the messenger. I only know that there is a compulsion to write it, the same compulsive force that led to our walk across Mid-America.

My primary desire is that you become active in managing your health. I am reminded of what a doctor once told me. He said, "If your doctor brushes off any question you have regarding nutrition or health care, without giving an educated answer or checking the science, he is either arrogant or ignorant." I agree with him, except I would add one other reason, greed. I've had an experience, and I'm sure I'm not the only one, where the doctor didn't even check what I went for, but chose to run tests for something that I might have at my age, but didn't. She was going to have a "suspicious" blemish on my skin removed that I've had for over fifteen years, but I wouldn't agree to it. The end result was she never checked anything to do with the problem I called her about, but I did incur quite a bill for the tests she ran. What was the motivation of this doctor? I'll let you be the judge but, in my opinion, the doctor did not have my best interests in mind and, therefore, I found it necessary to find a new doctor.

I am convinced that "living life to its fullest" means not only what you can do for yourself and others, but requires maximizing your health. You need all the strength and energy you can muster to enjoy your life and your interactions with others. So I want to express again that I believe it is in your best interest to take an active roll in determining what your "best interest" is. I think it is important to learn and know the latest scientific discoveries in cell-to-cell communication, because my understanding is that all diseases begin at the cellular level. AND all healing begins at the cellular level. Think about it! If two cells had not met and communicated, you wouldn't even be here. Can your doctor heal you? The answer is, "No." If you break a leg, can the doctor heal it? What he does, is provide a sterile environment and lines up the broken pieces. Then what? You wait six weeks as the body heals itself. Did we need the doctor? Of course! Someone had to know how the pieces line up and how to cast them.

What most of us do is manage our sickness or disease, or more aptly I should say deal with our symptoms. We go to the doctor for a prescription to stop our pain. It may eliminate our discomfort, but what I am asking you to do is to manage your health. Symptoms are the distress signals God wired into our body telling us that we have a problem. Masking or destroying symptoms is like seeing an army of enemy soldiers sneaking across the horizon; but since we don't want to think about it or feel it, we turn our backs, chug down some pain killers and pretend that they are not there.

We may be able to kill cancer cells with chemo and radiation therapy, but that does nothing to address the problem that allowed the cells to mutate initially. If you are still alive, you have some healthy cells that can be managed, even if you have a very debilitating ailment. Feed the healthy cells that remain and support their growth. Our bodies need not only vitamins and minerals, but also necessary monosaccharides (glyconutrients), essential fatty acids and amino acids. All of these are necessary for healthy cells. (Have you heard me say that before?) Check it out for yourself, by research or experiment. Our walk started with one step and did not finish until we'd taken 2,532,495 more (according to my pedometer). A return to health also starts with one step. That first step is always the hardest, making the choice to begin. Start by adding the proper fuel to build healthy cells and exercising to the extent you are able. As you build your healthy cells, build your hope.

If your blood pressure is too high, your cholesterol is elevated, your blood glucose is above healthy limits, etc., it may be necessary to take a prescription drug to lower the readings. But don't leave it there; don't accept it as a permanent situation. Get involved with your health management so you can decrease or discontinue that drug as soon as possible. Remember, all medicines have an LD 50 rating. LD stands for "lethal dosage," which means the drugs are toxic and, at extremely high dosages, can kill you. The maximum dosage levels were determined so that doctors would not prescribe them at a level to cause death. I'm not suggesting that you discontinue medications without your doctor's advice. I fully appreciate the doctor's knowledge; without their training, our lives would be catastrophic, if not disastrously short. However, I am suggesting that toxins are toxins. When you consume them, not only one prescription, but maybe five or six or even more, the increased level of toxicity combined with poisons we encounter in our environment (such as smog, auto exhausts, cigarette smoke, etc,) can do severe damage to your cells.

Get involved with managing your body's health, get serious about nutrition and exercise. Get adamant about minimizing stress in your life and removing fear, anger, and bitterness, one day at a time. Eat a diet containing several servings of fresh, uncooked fruits and vegetables, and add food supplements. Keeping fit can help you move mountains. Remember, the foods we eat today do not contain the same level of health benefits as we used to get. Food supplements should be a permanent addition to your diet, not stopped when you feel better. They should be included on your grocery list. Are you going to quit eating? Then eat food that will help promote cellular health. Recently, it was reported on TV that scientists now believe that table sugar is a bigger threat to our health than tobacco smoking. I also heard a doctor speak who stated that table sugar is one of the principal causes of ill health. "However," he continued, "there are necessary sugars without which you have virtually no hope for good health."

My personal suggestion is, curb both table sugar and tobacco. Did you know that when you "Super Size" your soft drink, you are drinking approximately 28 teaspoons of sugar? Yes, I said twenty-eight! Is it any mystery why we have the most obese population in the world?

Since Ron and I experienced the overwhelming improvement in our quality of life, I have been studying the glyconutrients and I am convinced that they are the first product a person should supplement into their diet. If your cells do not have glycoprotein receptors for communication, they cannot fully identify or utilize other good foods or supplements. Neither can they identify bacteria or mutated cells. God created our bodies to identify good and bad input through our cellular system, just as he created us to recognize good and evil actions through our mind and spirit.

What are your experiences? What have you learned from them? Will you share with us and others who need what you have … what only you can give to a needy world?

Epilogue
The End of This Chapter of Our Lives

I considered naming this chapter after Paul Harvey's signature quote, "And now, for the rest of the story---," but we don't know the rest of the story. As the picture on the front cover of this book so aptly displays, we can see where we have been, the ups-and-downs and the turns that we have already been through. But the road ahead is an unknown. It could be a challenge, it may be an adventure, and in most cases it will probably be some of both.

Have you ever known someone who pans for gold? First, he did his research to locate the most likely place to find the desired metal. Then he made inquiries to find what tools were needed to sift gold from the dirt, using the water. Once that information was established in his mind, he purchased the necessary gear and headed for the pre-determined destination. None of this is done without first conceiving an idea. Once that idea was birthed and the plans made, he launched upon his adventure. Is he surprised when he finds that shiny nugget? No, he went expecting to find it. Happy, yes, but not surprised. BUT suppose he doesn't find it after a few days. Does he quit? Does he throw away the equipment and refuse to search any further? Maybe … maybe not. But, let me tell you one thing I know without even one doubt. If he quits, if he refuses to search further, he will <u>never</u> find his treasure. His dream will fade and he will lose his hunger for the adventure.

Recently, I heard Pastor Steve Collins of the North Pointe Church here in Richardson speak on reaching your full potential. A couple of points he made were, first, "Speak life changing words. Avoiding negative talk is not enough; you must get on the offense and speak the blessings of God." Secondly, he said, "Speak blessings. With your words, you have the ability to help mold and shape the future of anyone with whom you have influence. A blessing is not a blessing until it is spoken. Words cannot be taken back. Choose to speak blessings over your life, your friends, your family and your future."

He closed with this scripture from Deuteronomy 30:19:

> *"Today I have given you the choice between life and death, between blessings and curses. I call on heaven and earth to witness the choice you make. Oh, that you would choose life that you and your descendants might live."*

Let me assure you that one day, life on this earth will come to a close. We may be granted rest from the trials of this land after challenging an extended battle, or we may leave quite unexpectedly. Let me ask you to live today, experiencing every good thing possible, as if it were your last. Whether you are struggling or whether you are walking on the mountain tops, live life today; we have no promise of tomorrow.

Now, in closing this chapter of my life and this book, let me speak a blessing and a prayer for you:

> "Today, I pray that you are blessed with a new hope for your life and for the lives of your loved ones. I do not know what your challenge may be, but I pray you will now become the challenger. You will look beyond your circumstances and into the adventures of your life, whether it is an unfulfilled dream you have decided to complete, whether you have decided to make changes that will reduce the anguished future of an obese child, or whether it be looking into the eyes of your caregiver and seeing for the first time how truly blessed you are that you have someone who is on this journey with you. Or maybe you are the weary caregiver, one of

those that I believe God holds in a special place in His heart. Whatever walk you are on, I pray you will take time to look at and listen to the beauty of God's creation, the flowers, the trees, the birds and animals, and find joy in discovering how intricately they are made."

Are not two sparrows sold for a penny? And not one of them will fall to the ground without your Father's will. But even the hairs of your head are all numbered. Fear not, therefore; you are of more value than many sparrows. (Matt 10:29-31)

I pray that your life will be an adventure and, at this moment, you understand that God has chosen life for you. God made you with great expertise, you were made to seek life and life is everlasting.

For God so loved the world that he gave His only begotten Son that whosoever believeth on Him shall not perish but have everlasting life. (John 3:16)
Amen

About the Author

First time author, Dorothy J. (Koenig) Martin, was born in a small community near Akron, Indiana. There she spent the first 57 years of her life before moving to Texas. In 1954, at the age of 16, she married Ronald Martin, who was 17 years old. Dorothy had continued her education after becoming a high-school drop-out. She received licenses in cosmetology and real estate and studied accounting to prepare for the bookkeeping and tax needs associated with her husband's service station business. However, it was not until she was 58 years old that she made the decision she was not going to complete one more job application, stating that she had not finished high school. Immediately she fulfilled that promise by going to the library, checking out the GED manual, and after studying the contents, tested for, and successfully passed the exam.

In 2004 Dorothy, with her husband Ron, walked from Dallas, Texas, to Akron, Indiana. This challenge was made to celebrate their 50th wedding anniversary after Ron had overcome a disabling bout with arthritis. To keep friends and relatives abreast of their whereabouts and well-being, a website was created. It was after the prodding from readers of the "website diary" that Dorothy agreed to write her first book titled *Challenging the Road Ahead*.

Dorothy is quoted, "If you are harboring a passion inside but feel incapable of completing the task, find someone who knows what you lack and let them help complete your "shortfall" areas; dare to seek and pilot your destiny." Dorothy's recent work as a bookkeeper for a non-profit Christian film review magazine, among other clients, brought her in contact with writers, editors, and fund-raising entrepreneurs who helped shape her dream of sharing her unique vision with others.

Printed in the United States
106453LV00003B/114/A